Mother Lode

Mother Lode

*Confessions of
a Reluctant Caregiver*

Gretchen Staebler

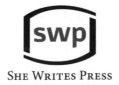

SHE WRITES PRESS

Published 2022
Printed in the United States of America
Print ISBN: 978-1-64742-283-7
E-ISBN: 978-1-64742-284-4
Library of Congress Control Number: 2022907328

For information, address:
She Writes Press
1569 Solano Ave #546
Berkeley, CA 94707

She Writes Press is a division of SparkPoint Studio, LLC.

Dedicated to my mother—the bravest person I know.
And to my father—we did our best.

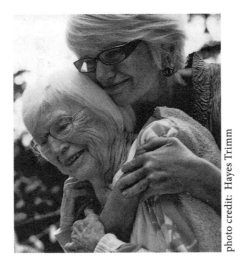

"By faith we travel to a land we've never seen by a road we don't know."

—Peggy Haymes

"Well, in that direction lives the March Hare. He's mad.
And in that direction lives the Mad Hatter. He's mad."
"But I don't want to go among mad people."
"Oh, but you can't help it, we're all mad here."

—The Cheshire Cat & Alice

Coming Home

As I prepare to leave for grocery shopping, Mama asks me to pick up some ground sirloin. "Be sure it's sirloin, I don't want ground round," she says, which I already know because she's told me a hundred times in the three months since I started cooking for her. "I like to have some in the freezer because I might want homemade pasta sauce. I don't like what comes in a jar. It's too salty."

"Did you like the sauce we had last night?" I ask.

"It was missing something," she says, after a moment of silence, as if trying to think what might be the right answer. "Did you make it or was it from a jar?"

"I made it," I say. "What was it missing do you think?"

"Salt," she says.

She can't see my eyes roll.

the first year

1

July

Arrival

I cross White Pass from central Washington's fertile Yakima Valley, Mt. Rainier rising to meet me, and roll past Packwood, Randle, Morton, Mossyrock, Cinebar, Onalaska—the names of the tiny towns a little too familiar. I don't head for Interstate 5 at Mary's Corner; I'm in no hurry to arrive at my destination. I drive across Jackson Prairie and text Rebecca from Chehalis, Centralia's sister town and high school athletic rival—"Swamp Swamptown, rah, rah!"—to update my arrival time. "Be there in fifteen minutes," I say. I'm five minutes away, but I'm driving slower and slower.

I slink into town past the "Welcome to Centralia: Population 16,731" sign, a block from the elementary school where I was a sixth grader when President John F. Kennedy was assassinated. I gulp. *Good Lord, what have I done?* "Centralia: Population 16,732." I am returning to childhood: the small town, the people who never left, the house, my old bedroom, and my mother's need to mother. I let my doubts go on the open road; now I'm terrified.

Smudge, my twelve-year-old diabetic cat who had settled down and slept most of the way across the country, is on high alert, sitting on her haunches in the dog crate behind the front seats of my fourteen-year-old Honda CRV, looking out the windshield. She is oddly silent as we drive down the potholed street through the neighborhood at the foot of the forested hill I grew up on. Transformation has not reached this part of town on the other side of the tracks, and the houses are more dilapidated than ever. The tennis courts with their sagging nets near the site of the original elementary school—damaged irreparably in an earthquake two years before I was born—have grass growing in the cracks. The empty lot, where all that remains of the school are the cement steps, is a tangle of pink-and-purple sweet peas.

My younger sister Rebecca's upscale gift boutique is two blocks beyond, across the train tracks on the town side of the renovated historic railroad station, out of place among the overload of antique stores. At least the sleazy taverns are gone; most of them anyway. The city has made strides in improving the few blocks in the center of town: flower baskets hang from reproduction streetlights lining the main street, intersections have been bricked and beautified. The cosmetic attention helps, but still businesses come and go in the historic buildings, and there are always empty storefronts as shoppers stick to the outlet mall and the Walmart shopping center at the Centralia I-5 interchanges two miles west on the other edge of town.

I turn right at the former lumberyard where I used to go with my father, the faded orange building a motorcycle sales and repair shop now with Harleys parked along the curb. The house on the corner has a sofa on the front porch and icicle Christmas lights hanging from the eaves in midsummer. Smudge moans behind me, echoing my fear. *Danger ahead; go back, go back.* But there's no going back now. My stomach clenches.

I head up Seminary Hill toward my old new home, the excitement of adventure gone. I will the car and time to slow down as I pass the National Guard Armory where a Methodist seminary sat before my time and gave the hill its name; where I caught the school bus half a mile from home when I missed its early arrival at the end of our long driveway. Across the road is the hill where I went sledding every winter. I wonder if the town's children still gather there. It doesn't snow as much now. Climate change.

After passing a couple dozen houses around the armory, the road climbs to a nonresidential stretch of bigleaf maple and Douglas fir forest, curving upward toward my destination, three-quarters of a mile from town. Unlike the hill above the hospital on the other side of town, this one never met its potential, which suits me fine, though it means few neighbors and friends. No one will be out walking in the morning, no one sitting on porches chatting up evening walkers. Not that I ever had that, but I dreamed it for my future. I'm stepping into someone else's life instead.

I had wanted to come back to Washington nearly since I left, but I didn't expect to come alone, and I surely never intended to live in this town again. Another wave of nausea passes over me. *Small town girl triumphantly escapes with husband to new life; quietly returns alone, tail between legs.* All I need is the dead of night.

I turn off the road into the driveway and stop the car, leaning my head back onto the headrest. This had seemed like a good idea. *What the hell was I thinking?*

Inhaling a deep breath and sitting up tall, I put my foot back on the accelerator. *It's going to be okay,* I tell myself. *Meroow,* Smudge says from the back; in confirmation or dissent, I'm not sure. We curve up the driveway past the first neighbor's house toward the second house, then make the left turn down the last stretch toward my mother's home hidden in the trees. I roll slowly past the apple trees in the neighbor's orchard, laden with green apples. The fence around the meadow on my mother's side of the driveway is weatherworn, as is the small chalet-style barn that once housed our pinto mare, Scout. The trail behind the barn is gone now, the land clear-cut by a nonresident owner after I left home. The acres are forested again; I could rebuild the trail, create something of my own. I get a jolt of excitement, briefly replacing my queasiness.

I slowly round the last curve to the sprawling mid-century modern house sitting below the level of the driveway, the narrow lush green valley farther below visible over the flat roof. Mama, Rebecca, my daughter Emma—who moved to Seattle after two years in the Peace Corps following college—and her girlfriend, Wynne, are in the driveway jumping up and down, blowing kisses in joyous greeting. I notice that Emma, who whacked off her beautiful curly hair in Africa, is sporting a new faux-hawk. At nearly six feet tall, Wynne towers above my tiny mother who is waving her outdoor walking stick—an old broom handle, her only concession to the instability of ninety-six years. Like Mama, Rebecca is tiny but mighty. I'm letting my short hair grow out, and it's the same jaw-length bob now as Rebecca's. She colors hers though, while mine is au naturel—nearly white by the time I turned forty, though not yet as snowy as Mama's. It may be by the time this gig is over.

They have all made a place for themselves here, and I don't know where I'll fit in. People confuse me for my sister. Even though she is half a foot shorter, we both look more like our mother than our father, and sort of like each other. Everyone in Centralia knows her. I was my own person in North Carolina, but here I will be Rebecca's sister and Stellajoe's daughter. I've left my Self on the other side of the country.

I stick my sunburned left arm out the window and wave, which strains the shoulder I injured when I fell at a crossroad's grocery store in Bumfuck, Arkansas a week ago. Turning away from them, I pull into the carport and sit looking out into the woods for a long moment, my hands unable to release their death grip on the wheel. I thank my old car for getting me safely here—in spite of a lost bolt resulting in a screeching belt coming down a mountain in the midst of a dust storm on a godforsaken stretch of Wyoming highway—then take a deep breath, open the car door, and step out to greet my family and this new adventure.

2

July

Leaving Home

"**D**id she ask you to come?" friends asked when I told them my plan to leave my independent life in the city—my beloved house, my job, my friends, my first grandchild—and move across the country to support my mother, still living in our family home. No, she did not ask. Neither did Rebecca, who had made her own cross-country return years earlier and was doing more than her share as our mother slowly declined. My wild Pacific Northwest roots were calling and I was ready to go. A year living with Mama—who had been pushing my buttons since adolescence—in the rural, conservative hometown I couldn't wait to leave thirty-six years earlier, was my rock to land on, briefly.

I hadn't made the decision to come home impulsively. I started plotting my return five years earlier, after the end of a second "forever" partnership. I had left a twenty-year marriage over a decade before when, astonishingly, I fell in love with a woman. Ten years later we separated too. I had promised "till death do us part"; divorce—legal or emotional—was not in my life plan.

In my midlife singleness, I had the best friends I'd ever had and a good job as an administrative assistant in a midsize church. I was living by myself for the first time in my life, and I loved it. I liked my adopted city of Raleigh, just not anything around it. I yearned for hills and valleys and someplace to go on Saturdays to get out of town and into nature for a few hours. I missed fir trees and rain, mountains and the wild coastline. I hated hot summers and looking out for copperheads and poison ivy in the garden.

One night, swaying in the swing on the porch of my tiny, rented house, the knowing slipped through me like the warm summer evening breeze: *I don't have to live out my life in central North Carolina.* I could return to my familiar, to where the air smelled damp and fresh. I could go in five years, I daydreamed, when I turned sixty. The idea was comforting, and it was a long time off. I could stop agonizing about it.

I bought a renovated craftsman-style house I loved. I grew confident caring for it and restoring the old garden. I visited my son and his family, including my grandson, when I could, though they rarely made the 250-mile trip across the state from Asheville to Raleigh. I briefly considered staying put. But as my birthday loomed into view, I revisited my promise to myself. I was getting itchy for a change. *Maybe leaving* is *who I am*, I thought. I liked new challenges. Maybe it was time to see what was around the next curve in the trail.

Though Mama wouldn't admit it, she needed me—and for sure Rebecca did. When Rebecca returned seven years after our father died of a heart attack the day after my forty-third birthday, Mama was still strong. Though past the midpoint of her eighties when Rebecca arrived, she had been capably, if obsessively, micromanaging a cadre of helpers to care for the aging 3,200-square-foot house and four acres. She didn't need much personal help other than to get to her many out-of-town doctors' appointments after voluntarily giving up driving due to her failing vision. In her mind, she was doing her youngest child a favor by giving her a place to live. When Rebecca moved to town and into the back of the building she had renovated for her retail business, Mama was alone again.

But the tide was shifting as I drew near my decade birthday. Mama was approaching the need for a housing transition herself, a fact she turned a blind eye to. Rebecca was juggling her business while continuing to eat dinner with Mama, sharing the cooking. Our elder sister, Jo Ann, also living on the eastern seaboard with her husband and his career, was not going to help. Did I feel an obligation, or did I just want an excuse to return to Washington? I couldn't work out the answer.

For the next few weeks, I vacillated between excitement and panic. How could I leave my son and his family—a second baby on the way? How could I leave my friends? How would I make a living, save for my own old age? How would I live again in the small conservative town? And the biggest question: How would I live with my mother when I could barely get through a phone call of her complaints about her health and her constant advice and worry about me—a holdover from her conviction that I had destroyed both my life and my children's when I divorced. Living three thousand miles apart, it had been easy not to have a real relationship with her, but now I was going to live with her? The questions nagged at me in the middle of the night, while by day I thought of mountains and fir trees and cooler summers.

I would stay with Mama for one year, I decided; twelve months of relatively expense-free transition time. Rebecca and I would get our mother settled in a new home, the house ready to sell, and then I would find a job and go back to my own life in some pleasing Pacific Northwest town—one I hadn't grown up in, one I could call my own.

With a good dose of terror, I offered to return. It was my ticket to

Washington; it was going to be fine. Wasn't it? Rebecca was ecstatic. Maybe she sensed a return to her own life. "Don't let me get stuck there," I said, and I made her pinky swear. It was only much later I realized my mother's response had been less than enthusiastic.

I committed to one year of a life interrupted—an older version of a gap year—and hoped I could stay in touch with my sanity long enough to fulfill my promise.

༄

Two weeks before I pulled into the driveway, I loaded my small SUV with a few clothes, a cooler with food for me and insulin for Smudge, the oil painting a friend made of my beloved house that I didn't trust to the movers, a used Rand McNally atlas with a tentative route marked, and my newly upgraded AAA Gold Plus membership card. The day after friends and co-workers threw me a party for my sixtieth birthday, I drove out of the city that had been my home for twenty-four years. Smudge—a black-and-white tuxedo cat shaped like a bowling ball—was none too happy in her crate, and we howled in harmony. Everything I owned was in a moving van heading across the country. The house I loved belonged to someone else. It was too late to change my mind.

Rebecca was at the other end of my journey, clearing her leftover things from the two rooms she moved out of five years ago in the basement of my mother's house, readying the space for me. Beyond that there was nothing to prepare me for what I was getting myself into. As the miles rolled away, though, I slowly let go of my grip on what I thought my life would be as I turned sixty and began to look through the windshield rather than the rearview mirror. I was ready for adventure.

I stopped for a few days in Asheville to visit Nicholas, Kristy, and six-year-old Max, and to welcome my three-week-old grandson, Ethan, to the world. I wondered if Nicholas felt like I was choosing his sister over him. His father and I divorced when he was an adolescent, and he withdrew from me, blaming me for the family disruption, at least in my imagination. While his father and I shared residential care of Emma equally, it didn't work for Nicholas, and he lived solely with his father, widening the gulf between us. With his marriage and a child of his own, our once-strained relationship had become cordial, if not close. Would my move crumble our fragile reconciliation? And these little boys. Would I lose them? My heart ached.

On the morning I left, I put Smudge back in her crate and turned to open the driver's side door as Max barreled toward me from the garage where they were waiting to wave goodbye, throwing himself into my arms for one more hug. "I love you, Gigi," he said, as I fought back tears. I drove down their long driveway to the road and waved back up the hill to him, standing alone, his parents and baby brother back in the house. When I was out of sight, I pulled off the road and wept.

A glass of water toppled into my laptop before I left Asheville, and it sat in a box of rice in the back of the car, my intention to blog across the country closed up with it. My cell phone's basic plan was for emergencies only, so I didn't text. I was alone on the open road in the middle of the country, my old life behind me, my new life not yet reached. I reveled in the adventure, the slow transition, and the off-the-grid silence before arriving in western Washington to begin life with my mother.

Like a pentimento—a trace of an earlier painting visible under one layered on top—I had layered several lives on top of my childhood. Scraping off the richness of those intervening years, I was home.

⌒∿

I hug Emma, Wynne, and Rebecca tightly, and Mama gently, afraid
of crushing her bird-like bones. They tell me they knew I was taking
pictures of the Burma-Shave style signs they had nailed on the fen-
ceposts as the car came haltingly down the driveway: YOU ARE
HOME. And I am, misgivings briefly set aside. I'm beyond grateful
that I will live again in the same state with Emma, that I will get to
know Wynne, whom I met a few years ago. However hard this will be,
there is that. Carrying Smudge, I follow them down the steps under
the arching overgrown rhododendrons and through the front door.
My panic returns.

The familiar musty smell of too much stuff kept too long in a
too warm house closes around me. I walk into the large living room
and put Smudge down on the stained beige carpet. The worn fabric
accordion shades on the five picture windows that extend across
the width of the living room are lowered, as are the venetian blinds
with bent slats on the adjacent triple-pane sliding glass deck doors
in the dining room. The light hurts my mother's eyes, one of them
permanently dilated from a cataract surgery gone wrong years ago.
I imagine the valley the covered south-facing windows overlook:
Mt. St. Helens—what's left of her—at the east end and the shopping
center between Centralia and Chehalis in the distance to the west.
There were no window coverings when I lived here before, and I have
never covered my own windows, but this half-light is what I have
returned to.

I scoop up shell-shocked Smudge before my mother stumbles
over her, while Rebecca retrieves her litter box and food bowls, and
the girls empty the car. We head to the basement and our quarters,
which Rebecca and I painted when I helped her move here. I returned

to my own home that time, weak with relief that I wasn't the one moving in. I'm grateful now for her colorful, whimsical style, a contrast to the tired ivory paint and brown paneling in the rest of the house.

There are no fresh daisies on the bedside table like there were when I came to visit in summers past. Later I will wonder if that was intentional or merely an oversight. Smudge sniffs around the kitchenless apartment with more interest than I feel, then retreats under the bed, from which she will emerge only for food for several days. I want to join her. I sink onto the bed, jolted by the realization that I will never again return to my childhood home for only a brief visit. It's where I live now.

It's three days after Independence Day; 365 days to go until I get mine back. A low rumbling growl comes from under the bed, and I take a deep shuddering breath.

3

July

The Wedding

The first two weeks following my arrival are spent in preparation for Emma and Wynne's wedding at Mama's home. Mama has a lot of anxiety about it, and it's my job and Rebecca's to keep her calm and reassured. She worries about the location of the port-a-potties and young children and dry vegetation around the gas grill and where the few people staying at the house will sleep and the strain on the septic system. She does not have anxiety about the fact that there is to be a wedding of two lesbians in the conservative small town where she is well known.

When Rebecca and I each divorced two decades ago and later Rebecca revealed that she was gay, our father was tormented. It was hard to untangle if he was more intolerant of homosexuality or divorce, which he found unforgivable. Although I never came out to him, he knew, and we hadn't spoken in the seven months before his death, so deep was our disappointment in each other. I wasn't home when he finally called me on my birthday and had not yet returned his call. He died the following day. We try not to believe his heart literally broke from disappointment in his younger daughters.

My father's pride in me, as a child and beyond, was of utmost importance. If he snapped at me for not holding high enough the end of the board while he sawed—*Dadgummit! Don't let it drop!*—I was crushed. When he praised me for the initiative I took in making a brick path without instruction—however poorly—I glowed. That he died disappointed in me, still angry even, has been a source of barely resolved grief. I wonder if I am here now magically thinking that if I take care of my mother I will win back his approval and his love.

I always assumed my mother let him dictate the depth of the wound and dove in with him. That after he died, realizing she needed her family, she sucked it up and embraced us as we are—gay descendants who now included my daughter and Jo Ann's son.

"Would we still be a family if Daddy were here?" I ask her.

"What do you mean?" she replies.

"Would we be having a wedding of two women here? Would he come? Would you be as accepting of your daughters and grandchildren?"

"Oh," she says, "I would have brought him around."

I'm speechless; it's not how I saw the balance of influence in their relationship. I have a hint of new respect for her.

༄

The big day arrives, and Mama is magnificent. She toasts the couple under the strings of lights in the yard after the ceremony, welcoming the eighty-five guests to her home, including Nicholas and Max, who have come from North Carolina, leaving Kristy and six-week-old Ethan behind. She welcomes her new granddaughter-in-law into the family, saying how much she loves Wynne and how perfect she and Emma are together. "I'm so glad she's mine," Emma tearfully tells me later. Me too.

∽

A few weeks later, prior to Election Day when Washingtonians will pass a marriage equality referendum, Mama gives an interview in our living room to the conservative local newspaper. From my perch on the stairs out of sight, I hear her speak eloquently and passionately for everyone's right to legally join lives with the person they love, beginning with a story I have never heard.

"I grew up in Tennessee knowing nothing about homosexuality," she tells the reporter, "but I did know about discrimination. A girlfriend and I attended a large Southern Baptist church across the street from my home. My family didn't have much, and we lived on the border of the white neighborhood and the Negro neighborhood. I was taught to cross the street when a Black person was coming toward me. But I learned a song in Sunday school that said 'red or yellow, black or white, we are precious in his sight,' and I came to believe we were supposed to love all people.

"Because of its location, our church had lost most of its members and was struggling financially. I gave a senior sermon my last year in high school, and suggested we invite our Negro neighbors to our worship service. It didn't make sense to me that the beautiful sanctuary was nearly empty every Sunday. After the service, no one spoke to me except my best friend. Not even the minister. We went to a different church after that."

"Do you think this referendum on gay marriage is like racial discrimination?" the reporter asks.

"People are born the way they're born, and they can't change that. I think the vote in November is about choosing between freedom to love and discrimination. I plan to vote for equality. My husband and

I were married for over fifty years, and I believe everyone should get to marry the person they love."

I sit around the corner, weeping. Her prejudices against so many people—smokers and the overweight, the homeless and unemployed—seem incongruent with her championing of this marginalized and persecuted group. But perhaps it goes back to her belief that those other people could and should fix themselves, while homosexuals, like people of other races, are made by God and beloved by God as they are. She is not just my mother, I realize; she is Stellajoe Staebler, community activist, and she is mighty.

She gets a half-page spread in the same edition of the paper in which they publish my guest commentary on marriage equality. I crack open the door a bit on this mother I've locked out for so long, and let a bit of my heart in.

4

August

The House

Settling into my old new home is not so much a process as a yielding to status quo. The house is Mama's compass, her map of the past: nothing shall be moved or removed, whether or not she uses it. I visit my incarcerated goods, padlocked in the storage unit at the foot of the hill, bringing some little thing back to the house with me each time. I retrieve my stemless wine glasses, thinking if the dishwasher doesn't feel so different to her when she unloads it, she won't judge me for my glass of wine with dinner as she has in the past. The daughter of an alcoholic father, she's a lifetime teetotaler. I understand her lack of experience with moderation, but I'll need wine to get through this year.

I am in subterfuge training as I develop the skills to make my living here more tenable in a way she might feel was her idea, or without her knowing I've done it. I put my Cuisinart pots and pans in the back of the cupboard behind her battered Revere Ware and drag them out to cook dinner. I squirrel away my marble rolling pin, leaving her featherweight wooden one from my childhood gathering dust next to the dented tin flour canister with tomatoes painted on it that's been in use my entire life.

To make room for more of my things, I secretively move unused items from high kitchen cupboards she can't reach to the basement storage room that was my father's workshop until he built a new one over the carport after he retired. I push open the door, salvaged from somewhere, not quite fitting the frame and still sporting the tin "Stupidvisor" sign my sisters and I gave him for Father's Day decades ago. I cram things into the built-in cabinetry stuffed full of other never used or no longer needed kitchen equipment, boxes labeled "war memorabilia," stacks of handmade picture frames and artwork never put on walls, gifts my mother had no use for but won't get rid of because they were gifts, Rebecca's stored belongings, and boxes small appliances came in.

I shut and latch the cupboard doors and lean back against them. Closing my eyes, I hear the buzz of the homemade table saw and smell the pointed mountain of golden sawdust. I see my father in his clear safety goggles, a flat red carpenter's pencil behind his ear, lips squeezed together in concentration as he pushed a board over the blade. I hear the click of the switch when he turned off the saw, and the whir of the slowing blade. Taking a deep breath, I shut the door on what is over, pulling it until the loose latch clicks into place.

∽

Though the house hasn't reached a level of pathological hoarding, accumulation clashes with my need for a Zen-like environment, and the battle is on, even as I know I will lose the war. My father's compulsion to save came with organizational skills; my mother's compulsion does not. She saves paperwork because he did, but she doesn't know why, and she doesn't have a filing system that makes sense to anyone except her. Old letters, lists, and notes written on scraps of paper are stuffed in the cubby holes of desks upstairs and down. The filing cabinet contains years of paid bills, outdated health plan descriptions, owner's manuals for long gone appliances and power tools, my father's tax returns for every year since 1938, and detailed records of work done on the property since the house was built, along with copies of letters of complaint about the work. There are duplicate printouts of side effects of all the drugs she has ever taken. She asks for them at the pharmacy with each refill or when she has a new symptom she blames on a medication she's taken for years. I look up her questions on the internet now, but she trusts the pieces of paper because they "came from the pharmacist."

Bank statements and canceled checks are bound in rubber bands on a shelf in a basement bookcase. I fill a large box for shredding, then find years more in a cabinet. I'm sure she's never needed those statements and hasn't opened the cabinets in years, but a week later she confronts me, her voice dripping with accusation.

"What did you do with the shoe boxes of old checks on the counter in the family room?"

"I put them in a box to be shredded," I say. "Did you need them?"

"They are mine, Gretchen."

"I thought they were a fire hazard." I shrug as she walks away.

It will only be after she is gone that I speculate the saved and filed paper was proof that she was taking care of things in her husband's absence, doing what he did before the age of electronic records. She was a bookkeeper and a secretary long before I knew her, and a good one. She returned to that version of herself.

～

My history in crafts still decorates walls and display surfaces: the cross-stitch wall hangings, the crewel pillow, a wheel-turned sugar bowl and creamer, a photo lap quilt, a fabric-art box, leaf-stamped slab clay creations I helped my children make to gift her at Christmas. My own three-year-old plaster handprint hangs beside the dresser mirror in the master bedroom. I'm surrounded by my past with no power to stuff it away and live in the present.

The spaces my father once occupied—the workshop over the carport, the little barn, the tool and garden shed with two canoes still hanging at the side—echo with the memory of his presence, while the house is nearly void of him, filled with my mother's sole occupation since his death. Even in life, only his study—transformed from Jo Ann's narrow bedroom when he retired—was his. One long wall is covered with wood and brass award plaques and framed certificates from his illustrious forestry career. A four-drawer legal file cabinet and the huge desk he brought home from his office when he retired fill the end of the room opposite bookcases full of his books. The long desk drawer still holds the rubber stamps and the drafting tool set he bought in postwar Germany that I played with when I visited him in his office. I sit in the executive-sized chair and swivel around as I did when my feet didn't touch the floor. Other than my mother's additions to the files, the room is as he left it seventeen years ago.

When I need to spend time with my father now, I kick open the swollen door of the "new" workshop over the carport. My family came the summer of 1989, and along with my father's brother and friends, we had an old-fashioned "barn raising" to erect his dream shop. By the time he built the interior, he didn't have much time left to use it before he died. The room still smells of Douglas fir and turpentine, and of the emptiness of his too-brief time here. Screws fill Gerber's baby food jars on shelves he specially made for them; nails of all types fill Darigold half-gallon milk cartons—the only brand my mother has ever bought—cut down to perfectly fit the shallow drawers in the workbench. Dull carpenter, hack, and coping saws hang on nails on the wall, and cans of crusted paint sit on shelves. His hard hat and red surveyor's vest—a sighting compass still in the pocket—hang on a coat rack, and his last pair of leather gloves lie on the end of the workbench. Scrap lumber is secured along one wall, a drill press and lathe sit at the back.

Rebecca used the space for her painted reclaimed furniture enterprise, and her paints and other tools of the trade are squeezed among my father's things; thrift shop furniture that will never be refurbished fills the corners and hangs on hooks from the ceiling. Boxes packed with her belongings when she left Maryland are stacked along the walls. I take over the small room at the back for a writing and crafts studio. I want to live here and leave the house to my mother.

⌯

I'm free to do whatever I want in the basement suite Rebecca fancifully painted. After the living room and bathroom were finally drywalled and finished in the 1980s as living space for my mother's mother—who refused to live there, objecting to life in a basement, feeding my mother's ongoing guilt about not caring well enough for her mother—it remained unfurnished but for cots for visiting grandchildren. But I don't think to make changes; Rebecca has impeccable taste.

When my father drywalled and finished the attached bedroom when I entered junior high, I had a room of my own for the first time. It was not kept as a shrine after I left home, and now nothing in it is mine. I sleep in the iron-frame double bed Rebecca left behind. The small desk in the corner was my mother's before she was married. The mirrored antique dresser, acquired after I left home, replaced the one that had been my parents' first dresser that I took when I moved across the country, a single piece of furniture with which to start my own first home. A lonely lover, it lives in the storage unit, waiting for me to come back to it.

I lie under the quilt I made for my bed under the eaves in my little home in Raleigh and fall asleep to the *who-whoot-who-whoo* of a barred owl through the open bedroom windows. In the moonlight, the coyotes howl in the forested hills.

⌘

I awake at first light and gaze out at the fog that fills the valley, hiding the rundown mobile home park on the valley floor and the red barn halfway up the hill on the other side. The trees beyond my curtainless windows are ghosts below the fog line, their tops glistening in the rising sun as the sky turns pink behind Mt. St. Helens on the eastern horizon. Mornings like this were my favorites when I last inhabited this room. I feel above the fray, just me and the sky. I breathe in happiness to be back to it.

Bang! I bolt upright in bed, my heart pounding.

The clock says six, but I know that without looking. At this hour every day, the oil furnace in the laundry room next to my bedroom comes to life, its metal housing expanding when the heat hits it. Obviously I'm not used to it yet. Mama's frail eighty-pound body is always cold, and the thermostat is set at 78° during the cool Pacific Northwest nights. When the afternoon temperature reaches the nineties and the sun hits the southern exposure wall of windows, she opens the deck door and turns on the box fans to move the hot air around. For a while, I turn the thermostat down and tell her to put on another sweater, then give it up. I learn that a symptom of dementia is an inability to tolerate discomfort even for a moment, and I start getting up at five o'clock before the furnace cranks up so I can wrap in a blanket.

I lean back into the pillows and listen to the calves bawl in the pastures hidden in the fog far below me as they are wrenched from their mothers to be weaned. I imagine them pressed against the fence, their mothers so close on the other side and so unattainable. I wonder if the mothers are relieved to be done with them, and what their reaction would be if their children returned, crushing their mothers' liberation.

I fight not to disappear into the shadow of this house that is where I live, but not my home; where the mother I have not known for decades fights to stay in control of her life and my father lives beyond death.

5

August

Last Stand Kitchen

"Put the forks in the back right corner of the holder in the dishwasher," Mama tells me, "or I have to rearrange them."

"Why?" I ask, determined to relieve her of her obsessions.

"Then I know where they are, and I won't stab myself when I empty the holder."

"So you can see to rearrange them, but you can't see them when you put them away?"

Sarcasm has always been my undoing, but she moves on without taking the bait. I close my ears to her next instruction and drift into adolescent memory.

I glare at my mother from across the corner of the counter to where she stands at the sink, correcting my dishwasher loading. "What difference does it make?" I sneer. "They still get clean."

"Don't sass me, Gretchen! Go to your room and think about your attitude," she snaps.

"I'll go because I want to, not because you told me to," I hiss back at her, stomping down the stairs to my room. Slamming the bedroom door I throw myself on the bed. "I'm never going to talk to you again!" I scream into the emptiness. "And I mean it this time!"

The minutes tick off: one, two, three, four. I open my US History book and start answering the end-of-section questions. Suddenly I remember something that happened at school. Jumping off the bed, I fly up the stairs and burst into the kitchen. "Mommy! I forgot to tell you something!"

I regress to my teenage self at the speed of light. I expose my buttons in a stubborn refusal to give up my own independence, and she can't keep her fingers from pushing them. We stand in the middle of her kitchen fiefdom with all our ancient anger. I am sixty and she is ninety-six, and nothing has changed since we were fourteen and fifty.

I receive instruction on a variety of things that in forty years of living on my own, Mama apparently cannot believe I have learned. She shows me how to open and close the blinds, walks me through hanging a picture on the wall, and demonstrates that the sliding glass deck door has to be closed all the way before it will latch. She reminds me about the sensitive septic system, as if it's news.

It's in the kitchen, though, where she will make her last stand. She shows me where to hang the dish rag, the proper way to replace the wastebasket liner, and how to place the can opener in the drawer so the knob doesn't catch when the drawer is closed. I bite my tongue and don't suggest putting it in the adjacent deeper drawer.

Chastising me for putting a hot cookie sheet on the vinyl countertop, I snap. "It's on a rack! You can't see it because there is a cookie sheet on it!" But she has already moved on.

There was a time when I was contained, whole, within my mother; a time when I skinned my knee and went to her for comfort; a time when I woke from a nightmare and slid into bed beside her for safety. But those times before childhood's end are thin strands in my memory. My sassy adolescent struggle into adulthood and her simultaneous stormy menopausal journey into her own life transition are my remembered hormonal core of our adult relationship. My family didn't talk about emotions, so I was left to figure them out for myself. The conclusion I came to was that it was my surliness that caused Mama's frequent tears and the fights between her and my father, none of which I had ever witnessed before. I was in my thirties before I understood it was menopause; that it was her uncontrolled hormones causing the personality change, not my own hormonal adolescent rebellion—though I probably exacerbated it. Jo Ann had been a model teen five years ahead of me, but I was incapable of stopping my driving need to lash out whenever I felt crossed as Mama quickly took the upper hand.

I left her after that—college, marriage, a move across the country—and became my own person. The whole of the country stretched between us for the next thirty-six years. We entered an adult relationship that had little soil in which to grow, my divorce midway through sullying what connection there was. I'm back now, in her home, hoping it's not too late to repair the breach as she fades into dementia. She needs me now, but she is still the mother. And mothers care for their young, not the other way around.

◦~◦

When I was growing up, the kitchen was control-central, organizing my mother's life. She cooked for her family and prepared her three daughters for marriage, lessons mostly confined to properly cleaning the kitchen and making meatloaf, banana bread, and chocolate chip cookies. When her children left home, she spread out in the house and into the world, becoming Stellajoe Staebler rather than Mother.

Her world has shrunk again with the adult child take-over, and she's back within the walls of her kitchen. After my father died—taking with him his health issues she obsessed about, since he didn't—she began working overtime to keep up with her own ailments. Chief among them are her "belly" and what goes down her throat that might get stuck in a kink left from a mismanaged emergency appendectomy at sixty-one, or cause gas, or that she claims she's allergic to.

She spends most of her days preparing what food she can, storing and labeling leftovers she'll often forget to eat, clipping recipes she'll never use, looking for things I might have changed in her domain. I don't yet realize that her ability to keep control of that small room in the center of the house when so much else overwhelms her is what has kept her going well into her tenth decade.

Cooking dinner is my most important task; preparing the prescribed food in a way she can digest it, the instructions changing meal to meal. I can't do it with her hovering over my shoulder, much as she would like to be there keeping an eye on me. For a large house, built when the kitchen was not a gathering place but the lonely bailiwick of the "housewife," the kitchen is small. Being alone there with my glass of red wine and *All Things Considered* on NPR is my nonnegotiable. I kick her out when I need to start dinner. I hear her tell friends I won't let her in the kitchen.

∽

One evening, bent over digging through the refrigerator, suddenly I feel viscerally what it is like to be her: a woman used to being in charge of her kitchen being told by her uppity daughter that she has messed up, that she bought kale and turnips at the tiny farmers market with the patient Michelle—her one-morning-a-week helper—when there were already kale and turnips in the refrigerator. She enjoys shopping for vegetables, giving her the illusion of control over something when she has lost so much. I mentally remove her finger from the "you aren't good enough" button she pushed when she implied that she doesn't trust me to get "good" vegetables. My job is to use what's here, which means figuring out how the hell one cooks kale (bacon makes all things edible), chard (with goat cheese), and turnips and rutabaga (soup, for her). The internet is my friend as I try to become a five-star cook in a two-star kitchen.

This is her last battle. I will get my independence back, I remind myself, even if it feels lost now. Hers is leaking permanently away. *Drip, drip, drip.* Perhaps the endless instructions remind her that she is competent and lull her into believing that, as my mother, she still knows more than I do. That I know how to change a light switch in an electrical receptacle or replace the flushing mechanism in a toilet or use a power tool would never occur to her because she has never done those things. The kitchen was where she knew how to do everything better than anyone else did, and she isn't going to let it go. She doesn't tell me to stop sassing her, and I don't stomp off to my room, but I still lose every battle.

I swear when I am old, I will never step foot in the kitchen, except to get ice cream and wine.

6

August

A Walk in the Woods

I need to get Mama out of the house, out of the kitchen. She is still steady on her feet and she walks up the driveway by herself with her walking stick. A fall would be disastrous, but I haven't been here long enough to think about that. I'm just happy to have a few minutes of solitude in the house, and I suppose she is happy to be away from me so she can stop instructing. She is afraid, though, to walk alone in the woods—her happy place—with the roots and uneven ground. I don't know why she doesn't ask me to take her. I decide to suggest it.

"I don't think I can," she says.

"Why not?" I ask.

"I don't want to bother you," she says, as if the operating instructions are not a bother.

"Let's go," I say. "It will be fun."

She sighs, like she's agreeing to go for my sake. *Good enough,* I think, playing along.

We walk up the driveway and across the meadow along the fence that separates our former horse pasture from the neighbor's yard and onto the trail at the back of their house. Mama walks slowly ahead of me, pointing out with her broom handle where I should look for trillium in the spring and wild trailing blackberries in July. Her eyes are weak, and I wonder how she knows where she is; then I realize she knows this place by heart.

The woods are old and broken down here behind our neighbor's house. There are no large conifers on the land logged in the 1980s, as there are down the hill in the "park." Licorice fern grows in crotches of the moss-covered branches of the bigleaf maples with dying tops. Arching vine maple drip with lichen; knee-high sword fern covers the forest floor.

It's the woods I played in as a child, my neighbor friend and I pretending to be horses, galloping down the trail, leaping over logs. Later, when we both had real horses, we rode for hours here. Barbara's family moved away as I was starting high school, and I lost interest in the woods and the horse.

When my mother's family-raising duties ended, the woods became her playground. She and a friend walked the trails every week, down into the undeveloped park owned by the city water department, where they led Girl Scout day camps together. When a rumor circulated that the department was planning to sell the trees to pay for a newly-required cover on the water reservoir, my mother and her friend decided it was up to them to try to save them; no one else was going to.

My father the forester wanted nothing to do with their project. "Trees are a renewable resource," he pontificated; "they are meant to be cut and the land replanted." My mother joined the Sierra Club in response, an organization he loathed, and put a bumper sticker on their car—a defiance that was lost on me at the time. Her partner in opposition recruited her husband, and they pulled in the neighbor couple. The two men, according to Mama, talked my father into lending his respected name in the community to the cause. I think now it was also a case of keeping family harmony: my stubborn mother had made a decision, and she wasn't going to let it go. "He could join me or oppose me," she told me recently, "but I was going to do it." She didn't use the words "hell bent," but I could hear the sentiment.

The group formed a "Friends of the Hill" organization, gathered signatures on a petition, pulled in the mayor who won over a narrow majority of the city council, and first temporarily, then permanently, they stopped the chainsaws. The seventy-two acres are now an official natural area, to remain so in perpetuity. This is my mother's legacy.

We walk to Staebler Point, a clearing overlooking the reservoir that needed a cover and the city beyond where a marker proclaims my parents as "leaders in preservation." Only much later did I begin to realize what she had done and the courage it must have taken for my introverted mother.

As we sit on the log bench to rest and have a sip of water, I look into the tops of the towering Douglas fir trees around us and the realization of my mother's accomplishment pierces me. *This wouldn't be here but for her.*

"I'm so proud of you and this place," I say, my voice catching.

"I didn't do it by myself," she says.

"Nobody does anything by themselves, but it has to start somewhere, and it started with you."

She doesn't respond. I hope she's proud, but she would never say so.

∽

"Thank you," she says when we get back to the house. "I thought I would never be in there again."

"You're welcome," I say. "We'll do it again."

She will never ask to go, and each time I suggest it, I will have to talk her into it.

7

September

Excursion

We're heading to Olympia today for a routine Ear, Nose, & Throat visit, a thirty-mile drive up I-5. It's my first doctor visit with Mama since my arrival, and my first full day with her away from home. When I come upstairs, she is standing at the door dressed to go with the cane she uses when we go out in the car and her bag of essentials: the disabled person parking placard, a tiny bottle of water, vials of preservative-free lubricating eyedrops, a packet of tissues, her notebook for recording what the doctor says, her purse, five Bed Bath & Beyond coupons, two expired Michael's framing discount ads, a baggie of Gas-X and Pepcid. Later she will add an adult diaper, rounding out the Ten Essentials, but her body hasn't made that betrayal yet.

It's thirty minutes before we need to go, and I want to enjoy my second cup of coffee. "We don't need to leave yet," I say.

"You are just like your father," she says. "He always waited until the last minute." I would rather be compared to my father, but I am a solid combination of both parents: my father's quick temper and his sunny optimistic outlook; my mother's stubbornness and her comfort with solitude. And her obsession with punctuality.

"Really, I'm like you," I say. "I hate to be late. So I built twenty minutes into the departure time and we still have thirty minutes."

She says nothing as she returns to her chair in the living room.

∽

We are an hour early for her appointment with the ENT, so we go to Target first, where Mama continues her hunt for a new watch. The search has worn Rebecca out; she warned me against engaging in it, but I'm fresh blood. She needs a black-on-white face with bold numbers she can see. But a man's watch or a sports watch is too big for her tiny wrist. Expandable bands can't be made small enough. She can't manage the buckle on a stiff leather or plastic band.

"Why do you need a watch?" I ask. She has, after all, been doing without for a long time, since her eyes were no longer able to see the tiny face of the Swiss watch my father bought for her in Europe in 1946, before he shipped home after the war ended. "Do you need it to tell you when you are hungry? Or tired?" I tease.

She laughs. "Sometimes when I'm sitting in my chair and there's something I need to do, I have to get up and go into the kitchen to see if it's time."

"We could get a clock for the table by your chair," I suggest. No answer. Not answering seems to be her way of telling me I'm obtuse.

We miraculously find a watch she can see, with a grosgrain buckle band that is almost tight enough on the last hole. The turquoise band matches her wardrobe better than the coral one, but she says the numbers aren't as bold. "They are exactly the same," I say. We purchase the turquoise-banded one and, after not picking up some other things on her list because they don't have the right brand, we head for the doctor.

We pull into the parking lot and Mama says, "Now that I have a watch, I can see if I have time to go to the bathroom before my appointment."

I'm beginning to realize I should follow her example of remaining silent, but I'm far from putting knowledge into practice. "Or you could ask, and I would tell you we have twelve minutes." Silence.

&

After an uneventful ENT visit—the cheerful and funny Dr. Kim telling her very loudly there isn't much wax in her ear, for which she was blaming further hearing loss and is surely disappointed there will be no quick fix—we have lunch at the Oyster House on Puget Sound's Budd Inlet, a family-favorite restaurant since my childhood. She orders her usual seafood Louie. As I watch the fork move to her mouth, I know what's coming. "It isn't as good as the last one I had," she declares, as I mouth the words along with her. I'm pretty sure the previous one was with me last summer and wasn't as good as the one she had before that. What is it like, I wonder, to be constantly disappointed? I suppose she at least knows it's coming. I give myself a mental high-five for keeping my mouth shut.

After lunch—which will serve as dinner, meaning we can have soup tonight—we go to the farmers market. For the fifth time today, I unbuckle her seatbelt and help her out of the car. I hand her her cane and, persuading her to leave her bag of essentials in the car this time so I can carry the bag of produce we will surely buy, she holds my elbow for the slow walk from the parking lot. She used to walk faster than I did; the change flits into my awareness.

We wander up one aisle and down the other, she looking for crunchy butter lettuce—the only kind she will eat—and feeling for "good" peaches and green beans. They all fail her criteria, and her favorite bakery doesn't have a satisfactory sweet treat she wanted for her breakfast tomorrow. An hour later we return to the car with only a pint of plump luscious-looking blueberries, even though she pronounced the sample not as tasty as the small ones we tried earlier that she had declared not very tasty.

Our last stop is Top Food—a pleasant, larger city grocery chain that has all her preferred brands in one place—where we almost don't get everything on her list because, she says, she can get them at the grocery store at home. Meaning I can get them. *"No!"* I say. "We are here, and we are getting everything on the list!" I'm too exhausted to realize she probably is too. She falls asleep in the car on the way home.

∾

Back in my basement suite after dinner, I settle in with a book I found at the library on caring for the elderly. I immediately chalk up my first bit of education. Gail Sheehy writes in *Passages in Caregiving: Turning Chaos into Confidence*: "The elderly complain about food not prepared to their liking or the wrong brand because they're unnerved by a world that feels too big for them to manage, and they want both the comfort of the familiar and the relief of making it someone else's problem." I mentally thank Gail, and promptly forget the next time Mama complains about a meal.

∾

The day after our excursion, I take my first lifesaving hike away from the house. I pack my knapsack with my own essentials: bug repellent, sunscreen and lip balm, water and food, toilet paper, moleskin, a bear bell Mama gives me. I spend the day alone at Mt. Rainier, basking in sunshine, beauty, alpine air, and the exhilarating and grueling hiking that reminds me I'm still young—and why I came home.

Three hundred and five days remain. Rebecca and I haven't begun talking about what's next or how to get ready for it.

8

September

Food Fights

The refrigerator, like Mama, is bloated and constipated—all input, not enough output. Like many in her generation, food hoarding is a leftover trait from the Depression, as well as her hardscrabble childhood. She keeps two bites of broccoli, a quarter of a small sweet potato, three bites of salmon from which she says she can make half a sandwich.

I can't figure out her criteria for when food is too old to eat and when it's still good. She chastises me for suggesting throwing out a very black half of a banana that has been in the refrigerator for days. She feels it and says, "There is a good bite at the end." The next day I find it in the garbage, but it was her decision, which makes it okay.

When she puts a previously unopened bag of spinach in the compost because it "expired" the day before, I share an AARP story with her. She is a lover of information, as long as I am not the source.

"The FDA has been saying for years that the date on food is not an indicator that it can't be consumed, that it's meant to help grocers rotate stock," I read to her while I sit at the table waiting for her to finish dinner.

She doesn't say anything, so I continue.

"Americans throw out fifty percent of food that could be consumed."

She sits silently chewing for a moment, then says, "So is it okay to drink milk that has lumps in it?"

I have no comeback.

~

In spite of the time she spent in the kitchen during my childhood, I see in hindsight my mother was not a cook. It was the dawn of the era of convenience, belied by the double wall ovens in the original house design, the second oven replaced now with a microwave. I was thirty years old before I knew asparagus as something edible, having had only the slimy spears from the Del Monte can. We ate Chun King Chow Mein with the attached can of dry noodles; Bisquick, hamburger, and cheddar cheese "deep-dish pizza"; Jell-O with fruit cocktail; creamed chip beef on toast; and the occasional liver. One night when I was perhaps ten, faced with liver on my plate, I declared that if I was made to eat it, I would throw up in my plate. "Eat it," my father said sternly. One bite later, I fulfilled my promise, and we never had it again.

Her tastes now run to dishes much more labor-intensive than tuna casserole with cream of mushroom soup or opening a can of anything other than fruit—because it's easier to digest—and Rosarita brand refried black beans, which I doctor with garlic and spices, thanks to the precedent Rebecca set.

~

I drive to Olympia today—as I do each Wednesday on my "day off"—to shop at Top Food and stock up on medicinal wine at Trader Joe's. As I roll across the prairie under the open sky dotted with fleecy cloud puffs, along the tall fir-lined interstate, I breathe in a way I never could in the South. No matter how challenging my new life is, I feel like I can do it here in this beautiful corner of the country.

The drive is my favorite thirty minutes of the week. The whole day stretching ahead for writing, yoga, reading while I eat lunch. Breathing. It preserves my sanity for another week. Or at least for the day. I'm grateful Mama can be by herself, and I'm sure she is glad for the empty house.

I linger over coffee and a bagel at Panera Bread, writing my weekly blog post and listening in on the conversations of other regulars, until time for yoga where I luxuriate in the ability of my body to do forward folds and downward facing dogs, forgetting for an hour my mother's aging body and the inevitability that mine too will one day be frail. I eat my packed lunch looking over Puget Sound from a bench on the wharf and then go to the farmers market for fruit and a pastry for Mama's breakfast. I wander past the vendors without having to tell my mother what's available and wait for her to touch everything, trying to ascertain if it meets her mysterious qualifications.

As I leave Olympia, I round the bend toward the I-5 exchange and, as it does every time, the majestic presence of snowcapped Mt. Rainier sparkling on the horizon against blue sky reaches into my throat and snatches my breath away. For this, I left the flat, featureless North Carolina Piedmont and moved back across the country. I'm about to need the reminder.

༄

I unload the car and take the groceries into the kitchen, where Mama is lying in wait.

"I went to the farmers market," I tell her. I'm proud of my purchases, sure this time she will be pleased too.

"Did you get any good vegetables?"

I breathe deeply, and with measured calm say, "No, Michelle took you to the Chehalis market yesterday; I didn't think we needed any vegetables."

Mama gasps. "You didn't look for tomatoes? Always look for good tomatoes!"

I roll my eyes, which her poor vision prevents her from seeing, but say nothing.

Minutes later, while not cooking the dinner I had planned because she says she doesn't think she should eat even angel hair pasta today, I ask: "Where did these grape tomatoes on the counter come from?"

"The market yesterday."

"There are also grape tomatoes in the refrigerator," I say, hauling them out as if I needed to prove it.

Mama looks at them and gasps in disgust: "They are from . . . Safeway!" She can see when she wants to. I feel my blood pressure rising; I should excuse myself and go to my room, putting myself in time out. But I don't.

"And here's a big tomato that's going bad." I take it from the refrigerator and barely avoid slamming it onto the counter. Why should I get tomatoes when they're uneaten? She ignores me, picking it up a few minutes later.

"What's wrong with this tomato?"

"I just said it needs to be eaten. It has some bad spots."

As I finish plating dinner, she says, "I'm going to eat this tomato you were going to throw away."

"I wasn't going to throw it away!"

"You said you were."

"No, I did not say that. I said there were tomatoes that needed to be eaten. And you were chastising me for not getting more." I'm getting light-headed, a warning.

"I didn't say that."

I breathe deeply and respond with Buddhist calm: "You said I should have gotten some at the farmers market."

"Oh," she says, "I guess I remember saying that."

I will lose my mind.

∽

I make a late afternoon run to the grocery store, reluctantly heading to the nearest one, where we shopped when I was a child, Fuller Market Basket, though it's now Shop 'n Kart, with a *K*. Nothing about the store has changed since I left in 1970 other than the switch to scanning cash registers, the addition of a lottery machine and, recently, hard liquor. It depresses me and I avoid it whenever I can, but it's the store where dairy products must be bought since Mama will only use Darigold from the Northwest, not Safeway's Lucerne brand because, she has told me, it's from Switzerland. Of course the Popeye-brand baby spinach at Fullers is inexplicably not acceptable, so I get no spinach this trip. Mama will have to do without her daily leafy-greens requirement tonight.

When I get home, I put the 97 percent fat-free ground round I bought on the counter and go downstairs to feed Smudge, forgetting to take time to unlabel it. Rebecca warned me to remove labels immediately, the therapeutic lie that hurts no one and saves everyone. When I return to the kitchen a few minutes later to start dinner, she's waiting for me. "Rebecca gets ground sirloin at Top's in Olympia. There's some in the freezer." I know that, of course; I bought it. My sister is a vegetarian and hasn't bought beef in decades—and she's never shopped at Top Food. But since I am the one living with Mama now, Rebecca's star has risen. "Next time, if you let me know ahead of time, I can get it out and thaw it," she adds.

"Sorry," I say, avoiding her gaze, "I didn't know until I was at the store what I was cooking," *or I would have gotten it out of the freezer myself.*

"What you got may say 97 percent fat-free, but Fullers puts gristle in it. Safeway usually has better hamburger than Fullers." Did she get out her magnifying glass to study the label, or did her vision momentarily return?

Taking a deep cleansing breath and exhaling slowly, I calmly inquire, "Would you like something else?"

"No," she says, falsely bright, "let's try this. It looks pretty good. Did you get my half and half?"

"Yes," I say, my resolve to stay calm heading into meltdown, "that's why I went to Fullers, because you won't use dairy products from Safeway, where they allegedly have better meat." She says nothing.

After dinner, she says contritely, "That was the best hamburger I ever had. Fullers must have gotten a good shipment in for Labor Day." *Or maybe they were too busy to add the gristle.* I sigh, wondering why she can't say I did a good job cooking it.

9

September

The ER

I got the baby monitor soon after my arrival. Mama thought she could use the whistle that hangs on her bedpost if she needed me in the night, but I couldn't hear her weak puffs into it from the next room, let alone downstairs.

"How about this?" she said, banging the spare cane that leaned behind her bedside table first on the floor, then the wall.

"If you are in distress," I protested, "how are you going to get out of bed, pull the cane out from behind your bedside table, and have strength enough to bang it?"

"You can hear me through the register if I call," she said, ignoring my question about the cane. She hated to spend money on anything that wasn't her idea, which was not to say she resisted spending money.

"I'm getting a baby monitor," I said firmly.

"We had an intercom," she said, "so I could call George if he was in the shop. You could see if it still works."

"It's thirty years old," I said, "and it has to be wired. There's new and easier technology now." I got a monitor; a cheap one in case the idea didn't work. Pleased with myself for defiantly solving an issue, I put the transmitter on the unused bedside table on my father's side of Mama's early-American-style double bed. I set the receiver next to the clock by my bed, where I listened to it buzz and to her snore all night. It had yet to be put to the test.

∽

"Gretchen!"

I wake with a start and glance at the clock: 11:14. I'm groggy, not sure if I heard Mama calling me or not. I turn the monitor up and listen. I don't hear her soft snore.

She moans, then, "Grehhtchuuuun." I jump out of bed, knocking Smudge to the floor, unplugging and grabbing my phone on the move. I snatch my glasses from the bedside table and shove them on as I open the door and race up the stairs and down the hall to her room.

"I'm here," I shout, knowing she isn't wearing her hearing aid. "What's happening?"

"I think I need to go to the hospital," she whimpers, rubbing her abdomen and groaning. "My belly hurts. I might have stomach cancer."

"You do not have stomach cancer."

"My mother had it, Gretchen," she reminds me, her voice abruptly strong. "I know the symptoms. I didn't flush the toilet, look and see if my stool is black or bloody."

It's the middle of the freaking night and I'm examining poop?

"It looks completely normal," I report back. It's not the time to ask what she thinks the ER is going to do about stomach cancer in the middle of the night, and it's not her real worry anyway; it has always been her habit to go to worst case first. She moves on to her real fear.

"I must have a blockage," she moans. She's had bowel blockages before—presumably from scar tissue caused by the appendectomy—and I vaguely remember a hospitalization when I was home for a visit.

"You did have a bowel movement, though," I say encouragingly. I want to go back to bed, not to the emergency room.

"It wasn't easy and it took a long time," she says, detailing how she got it out. She grimaces again, writhing in obvious pain and dry heaving. Her face is pale and drawn; she looks so old. The giveaway, though, is she's in too much pain to tell me she has to go to the hospital in Olympia. She has a mistrust of the local hospital, where they first misdiagnosed her appendicitis and then mismanaged the surgery, and where my father died of a heart attack. She has no memory of the fact that she wasn't happy with previous Olympia experiences because nothing traumatic happened.

Hospitals are not good places for the elderly, and taking her there is not a decision I have any intention of making on my own. I call Rebecca while Mama derides me for "bothering her." "This is why there are two of us," I say. When Rebecca gets there ten minutes later, Mama thanks her sweetly for coming. Rebecca and I have a brief conversation over the bed with our eyeballs.

We aren't sure she needs to go, but we don't know what else to do, and we don't want to be responsible for mistaking the need. If her primary care doctor—whom I've not yet met—has a twenty-four-hour call line, we don't think to call. We bundle her up and get her into Rebecca's car. At least we can avoid the trauma of an ambulance.

∾

The perk that comes with arrival at the ER in an ambulance is you get right into a cubicle. Rebecca knows this, but I have much to learn. We sit in the waiting room in plastic bucket chairs. A toddler lies frighteningly silent in his weary father's arms. A pregnant teenager sits with her mother, doing level one breathing. It looks to me like she should still be at home. While we waited for Rebecca, I tried to get Mama to use the labor and delivery breathing technique I still use in painful situations, like root canals and talking to my mother. She cannot learn new tricks.

Mama's uncomfortable in her hard chair, and she is cold, but she doesn't complain. We wrap her in the blanket I grabbed on our way out the door. Perhaps the assumption that she will get help—and that we gave her what she wanted, the hospital—mollifies her. Her pains become further apart and, judging from her now silent grimaces, bearable.

When we finally get to a cubicle and Mama is lying down, I recite her medications list to a nurse for the second time—with Rebecca's prompts—including the only prescription she takes, for her heart and that I can't pronounce, prescription eye drops, and the over-the-counter drugs: baby aspirin; Pepcid; GasX; Senna, an herbal laxative; and Colace, a stool softener.

"How often?" the nurse asks.

The hell if I know, she self-medicates! "As needed," I say. Should I tell them she chews peppermint gum in bed at night, insisting it helps with gas? I figure death is going to come from choking on gum in bed. I'll be asked for the list three more times, and I make a note to put together a hospital kit with a list of meds to hand them—including, as we will soon have firsthand knowledge of, those she should not be given under any circumstances.

Mama gratefully accepts warm blankets but refuses pain and nausea meds for her now brief and intermittent symptoms.

"Why won't you take something for the pain?" I ask her in frustration and curiosity.

"If the pain is masked by drugs," she says, "no one will believe there's something wrong." She wants answers to unanswerable questions, not temporary relief.

A woman in the next cubicle is moaning, "Oh, God! Oh, God!" and vomiting every few moments. The toddler—in a cubicle now, no doubt being poked and prodded—wails. The pregnant girl and her mother are still in the waiting room. The ER represents a whole world beyond my experience.

Rebecca goes home to her warm bed with her cat so one of us will be rested when daylight comes. I have no escape. Though Mama is mostly quiet, she doesn't sleep, and neither do I. Not that I could have in the plastic chair. The nurse wearing scrubs printed with dogs turns off the blinding overhead light when I ask her to and brings me two pillows. I stack the pillows in my lap and bend forward over them, but it's hopeless. The monitoring machines beep, curtains are slid open and back in the cubicles circling the ER, voices summon staff over the intercom, Mama tells me she's cold and I get more warm blankets and tuck them around her.

I hear the doctor enter the room of the moaning woman: "So, all this vomiting from one little drink?" he says. I get the feeling she is well known in the ER. I peek past the curtain when I go out in search of water. She is thin, her long stringy hair tangled, and her layers of dirty clothes ragged. She is alone. When I return to Mama's bedside, I scoot my chair a little closer to her gurney and put my hand over hers, grateful to be here. I can't imagine her in this place alone, her husband long gone and her daughters all on the other side of the country.

❧

In the early morning hours, Mama is finally taken for an X-ray and the nurse reports that the ER doctor thinks there might be a small partial obstruction. The words I did not focus on are *thinks*, *might*, *small*, and *partial*. But it is a necessary diagnosis to get her admitted, and she will not be satisfied to be sent home without treatment. I'm grateful not to have to take her home until she feels better. Later Rebecca and I will fervently wish we had.

10

September

Delirium

Rebecca joins me in the hospital room the next morning with lattes. I catch her up on the night, then go home to feed Smudge and get a couple hours of sleep. I turn off the furnace and open the windows to cool the house, then fall into bed.

As my body relaxes, I drift into memories of returning to my home after work and letting go of the day's stresses. My mother is not waiting for me to get a meal on the table, or telling me how many seconds to microwave her cup of water (one hundred thirty-three—buttons she can find without benefit of sight). I can wear a sweater without having hot flashes, feel the sun on my face through the uncovered windows and the breeze through the open door. I can read while I eat.

When I get up, I let Smudge out of our quarters to explore. It's the first time we've been alone in the house for more than an hour since our arrival almost three months ago. Smudge wanders upstairs and bathes herself in a rectangle of sunlight. I sigh deeply ten times and don't wonder how Mama is doing. Rebecca is on duty.

❧

When I return to Mama's room after lunch she is sleeping.

"The doctor came," Rebecca tells me. "He doesn't see a blockage on the X-ray."

"Great!" I say. "So why are we still here?"

"She needs to poop before he'll discharge her."

I'm equipped now with a book and my computer to connect me with the outside, though in further insult to the hospital experience, both cell service and Wi-Fi are sporadic. When Mama wakes in good spirits and no pain, we walk around the hall looking at photographs on the walls depicting Centralia's history in hospitals, including the first one that became the seminary on our hill. She tells me stories of one of her childhood homes that was near a hospital.

I text Rebecca with an update, telling her about our walk and talk.

"Nice," she writes back. "Our conversation was her wondering what you threw out of the freezer when you cleaned it out together last week."

I send a laughing emoticon. I guess Mama's feeling better.

She is still under nothing-by-mouth orders and, though she is getting IV fluids, her mouth is dry. I go to the nurses' station to request the ice chips the doctor told Rebecca this morning she could have.

"There's nothing here about it," the nurse says, looking at the computer record. "I can give you swabs, lemon or plain, but she can't suck them."

"We were also told a second X-ray had been ordered. Do you know when that will happen?"

"That's not here either," the nurse says. "I don't know anything about it."

"Do you know when she will be allowed to eat?"

"No, sorry," the nurse says. The top of my head is in danger of coming off. I know it's not her fault—she wasn't even on duty when

Mama was admitted—but I'm frustrated. I turn on my heel and return to Mama before I say something I'll regret. I wish for the paper chart at the end of the bed so we could see that the doctor recorded what he tells us on his rare appearances, but even I know Mama can't poop if she's not eating.

Rebecca returns late afternoon and Mama insists we go home for the night. "I'll be fine," she says. I'm sorry she's in the hospital, and I am ecstatic to be home alone again. I eat pizza in the living room and watch TV while Smudge sleeps on the sofa beside me.

∾

I take the first shift on Sunday morning, arriving at the hospital at eight o'clock with a sixteen-ounce half-caff latte—an indulgent perk of this adventure. Mama is sleeping.

"She had a difficult night," the morning shift nurse tells me.

"What happened?" I ask, alarmed.

"The night staff reported that she woke up around midnight complaining of chest pain and having a panic attack."

She's always imagining her chest pains are a heart attack, but they don't know that. I don't say anything.

"They couldn't calm her and they gave her half a dose of lorazepam."

I don't know what that is, but I think nothing of it as I sit beside her reading my book and catching up on my friends' lives on Facebook. Bored then, I Google lorazepam and learn it is a high-potency antianxiety medication, muscle relaxant, sleep aid, and more. I'm glad she's getting a good rest.

When she wakes up two hours later, her speech is labored, and she can barely lift her arms before they fall back to the bed of their own accord.

Concerned and not wanting to leave her side, I push the call button.

"Can you tell me more about her night?" I ask the nurse.

"Her panic lasted a long time; she was hallucinating," she reads from the computer in the room.

"How long is a long time, and what did they do to try to calm her?" I ask.

"It doesn't say."

"Why didn't they call? It's why my sister's and my numbers are on the board, with instructions to call if there is a change!" I've passed yesterday's frustration and moved on to furious.

Mama becomes agitated and in garbled speech shouts, "*No!* I didn't want them to call you!"

"It's a difficult decision for staff," the nurse says, her tone conciliatory. "Do we honor the family's instruction or respect the patient's wishes?"

My control all but vanished, I argue, "If the patient is ninety-six years old and in an altered state, you call the family!"

Initially Mama is laughing and joking about her state of loopiness, but when it begins getting worse rather than better, delusional rather than silly, and in a state of rising panic myself, I call Rebecca to come. While I wait for her, Mama tells me, "They tried to kill me," looping with "I think I'm dying," and "I wish they would have let me die."

Her tongue curls to the back of her mouth, and she can't speak at all. We don't see how she can breathe, and at our urging she is given light oxygen. We don't know if it's for our benefit or Mama's. We become increasingly panicked and convinced we are losing her as she spirals down into craziness.

"It's just the meds," the on-duty doctor tells us when he finally shows up. No one seems concerned that she's getting worse, which makes us more distressed. "It will wear off," he says. "If she isn't better by four, we'll do a CT scan to rule out a stroke."

A stroke! He throws that out casually? What is wrong with these people?

The seed was planted in fertile soil, and by two o'clock we are as agitated as Mama. We insist on seeing the doctor who orders the scan early. Being in the CT tunnel unhinges her more. When we see her again, her panicked speech is indecipherable, her arms flail, her head rolls from side to side, her face is a mask of *The Scream*. Rebecca and I hold her hands and stroke her head, telling her it's okay with a calm neither of us feel.

❧

The scan shows nothing amiss, and by four o'clock her state begins to reverse as the doctor predicted it would. By evening she is herself, but upset by the experience. "I had a terrible nightmare," she says.

"Do you remember the dream?" I ask.

"They gave me three little red pills to try to kill me," she says.

It's the last time she says it was a dream. For months afterward, she tells friends, doctors, and nurses she was drugged. She will not be swayed by the fact that she was receiving nothing by mouth at the time and the lorazepam was administered intravenously.

We spend three days in the hospital and never receive any treatment for her presenting symptoms. She has been tested for stroke and heart failure, and did not eat for two of the days. They finally let her eat, she has a bowel movement, and we are sent home.

❧

"Advocate" was not a part of the job description I had anticipated, but if I am to be one for my mother, I need a better source of information

than WebMD. I do an internet search of books on aging and parental caregiving to add to Gail Sheehy's book and order *Bittersweet
Season: Caring for Our Aging Parents—and Ourselves* by Jane Gross;
the words following the dash sell me on the book. When it arrives, I
devour it with my yellow highlighter.

Gross writes that anecdotal evidence indicates "extreme behavior is an especially common reaction to hospitalization among the
elderly, and they become unglued psychologically and/or cognitively;
entering the hospital in what seems to be a fully intact state, only
to become delirious while there." And CT machines are especially
traumatizing for the elderly.

Hospital delirium, Gross says, affects nearly one-third of hospital patients over seventy. It can be triggered, among other things, by
not having one's hearing aids or eyeglasses—neither of which anyone
thought to give Mama, though I brought them with me from home—
or by medication errors or anesthesia. Of those who suffer hospital
delirium, 35 to 40 percent die within a year, a frightening statistic.

It's the beginning of my education.

11

October

Mini-Breaks

Late in the week after our hospital adventure, I walk up the road. Maybe fresh air and early morning exercise will help my cranky disposition. Mama is physically fine, but the ordeal has left her frail and needy.

It rained last night, and along with the scent of dry earth finally wet—*petrichor*, a word particularly useful in this corner of the country—I breathe in the history of myself. I pick an apple from a branch of one of the neighbor's trees that hangs near the driveway and bite into it. Its crunch walks me to the ghost of the little shed where Barbara and I and our little sisters waited in the rain for the school bus at the end of the driveway. A grove of already old firs has taken over our former neighbor's horse pasture, and the cherry tree I climbed isn't there anymore. I walk up the hill past the houses where I babysat children who are probably grandparents now, remembering riding bikes and horses here with Barbara. At the first curve in the road, where Scout would always turn and bolt for home if Barbara and Shadow weren't along, my cell phone rings. It's Mama. She can't see to measure her hot cereal into the water, and she needs me. I don't make it to the pretty house with the long, grape-arbor-lined driveway where the manager of the JCPenney lived, or to the dead-end road where the World War II bride from France who taught me French after school in third grade still lives, or the art studio of my father's boss's wife at the end of the road where I struggled through watercolor lessons.

Sighing, I turn and head back home, any elation at being freed from my stall collapsing. There are no tears; this is my life now.

❧

Like Scout and Shadow, Mama and I are tied to each other by an invisible elastic band, stretching only so far before reaching its capacity and snapping us back together. At night I listen to her jagged snore over the baby monitor that tethers her bedroom to mine. On a rare evening out with Rebecca and her friends, one eye is on my phone as the band stretches to its limit. I imagine her eating alone the dinner I prepared before I left, then moving to her recliner with a cup of hot water, where I'll likely find her sleeping when I return. I wonder if she's glad for the solitude or if she feels abandoned.

I feel guilty for wishing the end would come for her. And I'm not ready. Mostly I wish it would come before she becomes consumed with gloom. My father died too soon, but perhaps because I didn't see him often during his years of declining health, he lives on within me, active and witty. I already can't remember my mother younger than she is now.

❧

Rebecca offers to take Mama to Seattle for her glaucoma specialist appointment, giving me a much-needed break and putting off my flameout. Six hours, an extravagance. I select a Beatles Pandora station on my computer and turn it up loud, singing along to "Here

Comes the Sun," my personal college theme song in rainy Seattle when I played the 45 rpm record over and over on my Sony portable stereo system. Smudge hangs around the kitchen while I clean out the refrigerator, which I will pay for later when Mama wants to know where something is.

Rebecca texts from the examining room.

"Mama just told the doctor she was given an overdose of lorazepam in the hospital and it robbed her of her vision."

I raise my eyes ceiling-ward. "What did the doctor say?"

"That her eye pressure and her vision are better than they were at her last visit."

"Did that stop her in her tracks?" I ask.

"Nope. She said that's because she cut back on her blood pressure medication."

"What the hell?" I say. "She took the increased dose the cardiologist prescribed for one day before she decided it made her tired and went back to the original dose!"

"I wondered about that. He told her that wouldn't affect her eyes."

To be happy her eyes are testing better would deprive her of her lorazepam theory.

I sit in the sun on the deck catching up on email. I find a three-week-old blog post from a pastor friend quoting Thomas Merton. In his letter to Jim Forest—a discouraged young peace activist during the Vietnam war—Merton writes on how we have to come to terms with the idea that our efforts, no matter how sincere, may be "worthless." He reflects:

> *As you get used to the idea, you start more and more to concentrate not on the results, but on the value, the rightness, the truth of the work itself. . . . In the end, it is the reality of personal relationship that saves everything.*

My friend writes,

> *You show up with authenticity, embracing respectfully the inevitable differences in any relationship, staying unattached to specific results. If you can do this, let's say, 60 to 70 percent of the time, well, that's huge!*

My mother is a concentrated version of the person she has always been—both the parts that make me crazy and the courage I find so amazing. It is how she has lived, and it is how she will die. I wonder if I can accept it 30 to 40 percent of the time.

∽

Mama meets me at the kitchen door when I come upstairs to greet her.

"You don't understand how the low water pressure on the hill affects the dishwasher's ability to get things clean," she says without preamble. "I had to scratch something dried off a measuring spoon and then soak it."

It's not the first time she's told me this—though I've managed to keep quiet until now—but I am not a child, and this is not how I want to start a day. I break my vow to respect our differences.

"Good morning," I say, modeling how one should greet another. "You don't always get things clean either."

"I'm sorry; I can't see."

"It doesn't matter. I've not seen the need to point it out, and I wish you didn't." She doesn't respond.

Her need for control and her insistence on micromanagement have gotten worse as she has aged. The kitchen floor has to be scrubbed on hands and knees or "it doesn't get clean." She hired Stan, a patient man in his forties, frail from hard living and Lyme disease, to care for the yard and the floors. He was living in a tent on the edge of our property when I arrived, evidence of her incredible caring and generosity that sometimes overcomes her judgmentalism.

Though Rebecca received a monthly stipend when she lived here, there has been an unspoken agreement since I joined the household that I was not coming to be the housekeeper, but to make it possible for Mama to carry on in her home a while longer, primarily just by my presence for now except for cooking. I was very clear that I was not to be paid. I would rather live frugally than be given a list of tasks and followed around to be sure I did them "right," followed by one of the periodic evaluations I find in a file for Rebecca.

I'm in desperate need of a coffee shop escape. After the dishwashing admonishment, I offer to strip Mama's bed and get a load of laundry going before I leave.

"No," she says, "I need to get my breakfast."

"That's fine," I reply. "I will do this."

She tells me where to put the blanket (on the guest bed) and the lap-sized comforter (in the study because it's too dirty to put on the guest bed). Then she starts removing a pillowcase.

"I am not going to stay and do this, if it means you won't go get your breakfast!" I snap. I am completely exasperated, and it's only eight in the morning.

She goes to the kitchen without another word, leaving me feeling like Worst Daughter Ever, again.

I put the load in the washer and tell her I'm leaving.

"How much detergent did you use?" she asks. Apparently we aren't done with morning lessons yet.

"A scoop full," I say, though I don't really know.

"You only need three-quarters of a scoop for a medium load," she says.

"Fuck," I mutter. I tell her I will do better next time and flee.

∾

Day 90 of 365. I'm like a prisoner chiseling hash marks on the walls of the cell. But she's the one walking the Green Mile. I will be freed. Someday. It's going to be a long, cold, lonely winter.

12

November

More Food Fights

Mitigating Mama's stomach and bowel issues via menu choices, in combination with her failing taste buds and high expectations, is as impossible as controlling the rain in November in the Pacific Northwest and daily drives me to consider early drink. It's been a typical week.

Mama's upset with me for throwing out a fifteen-month-old container of frozen vegetables from a friend's garden, half full of ice. "I had nothing to make soup with yesterday," she mourns when she discovers it in the garbage where I tossed it after we defrosted the freezer together. It was still in the freezer when she made the soup, but I say nothing. Some days I'm smarter than others, or more tired.

As apology, I offer to make the squash, turnip, and rutabaga soup for which we bought ingredients at the farmers market last week. She agrees, but she doesn't know where the recipe is. After looking through her vast collection of soup cookbooks at her insistence, I find one online that can be adapted. We spend ten minutes discussing the amount of spices to use: far less than the recipe calls for.

For the next two hours, prior to cooking dinner, I make the soup rather than doing the writing I had planned for today. I'm not a soup fan, but the few bites we have as a dinner appetizer are tasty.

"What do you think?" I ask hopefully.

"It's a little bland," she says.

I sigh.

Constipated again, Mama has requested tuna casserole for dinner, thinking she might be able to digest it. "But without noodles," she adds, "or cheese." *Is that even possible?* Although I succumbed to the cheap draw of tuna casserole as a poverty-level newlywed, I haven't had it for thirty years. I haven't missed it.

After I fail to find a recipe on the internet that meets requirements, Mama finds one in her *Chicken of the Sea: Tempting Tuna Cookbook*, published in 1976—when I was that young newlywed. The paperback book with plastic spiral binding is falling apart and is married to a brittle-paged *Joys of Jell-O* cookbook in a plastic Ziplock bag so the pages won't be lost.

I make the casserole to her specifications: tuna and white sauce baked with buttered breadcrumbs. I make pasta primavera with shrimp for myself.

"I need for you to tell me in the morning what you are planning for dinner," she tells me as I carry our plates to the kitchen after dinner. "Then I can tell you if I can eat it or not depending on how I feel."

I blanch. I had begun to feel like I had a handle on my terror of cooking for someone else every night again and was pleased that thinking about it was no longer consuming my day. I keep my mouth shut. We'll sleep on that one.

By the time I go to bed, I'm obsessing over what to have for dinner the next night. It's the first thing on my mind when I wake up. I have to come up with a solution to meal planning, or I will go out of my mind. She doesn't mention it again, but I know the bomb is ticking.

Two days later, in an attempt to give her more control over meals, I present her with a list of ten of her favorite entrees and ten side dishes, telling her to choose what she wants. Every morning she can assess her needs and pick her menu; her daily requirement of cooked greens and canned fruit provided as always. Pleased with my innovative approach, I say, "I'll make whatever you want, but I don't want to discuss it." Discussing food is more tiring than cooking it.

We try it for a few days, each day involving a lengthy morning discussion. I go to the grocery store every day and get the freshest ingredients. By evening she doesn't think she can eat what she chose.

On the fifth day—five days in which I have done nothing but deal with the evening meal—I'm ready to assess the plan. "This isn't working, is it?" I ask.

"I should have taken that best room at Colonial Residence when it was available," she says. It's a refrain she pulls out when things aren't going well. She's been on the waiting list for years for a specific apartment in one of the assisted living facilities in town, the director calling her when it opens up, she telling them she isn't ready. They called a few months before I moved home, and Mama called me.

"Are you really going to come and live with me for two years?" she asked.

"One year," I said firmly.

"So I should turn down this apartment?"

"Do you want to move there," I asked, "or stay at home?"

"If you aren't coming, I need to take it while it's available." It wasn't my question, but I let it go. Maybe I shouldn't have. Maybe she wanted to move.

"I'm coming," I said.

"Okay," she said, after a pause. "I won't take it."

My sisters and I went on a secret reconnaissance visit last time Jo Ann was home and talked to the director. Now I present Mama with a finding. "Are you aware that at Colonial Residence, you have a choice between two entrees, and you have to make the decision a week in advance?"

"There is a kitchenette in the room," she says, "with a microwave and a refrigerator."

"Are you going to cook every meal for yourself? If that's your solution, you can cook your own meals here in the microwave and save yourself the move *and* having to eat what I cook."

Her face shuts down.

I hate myself for being snarky, for failing to understand how hard she's trying, for falling off the edge of tolerance at her lack of appreciation of how hard *I'm* trying. And why am I discouraging her from moving? It's a question for which I have no answer.

13

November

Losing Control

As autumn slips quickly toward winter, the days grow short, the fog rolls into the valley on a daily basis, and the drought ends. Mama and I begin settling into an uneasy routine. I become a little less derisive and a little more accommodating and understanding. It's slow going, and I regress over and over, allowing myself to be pulled into her web of anxiety and need for control.

I begin to see our connected lives like the intricate path of a labyrinth. My mother is spiraling inward toward the center, the still point of the turning world. Someday she will be unable to care for herself, unable to find her way back out. I am following the outward way toward assuming the reins of care, trying not to step over the bounds of the path in front of me. I walk outward toward my own freedom, then turn back toward her. She approaches the center, only to depart from it again. Occasionally, as we pass close to each other, I have an inkling of understanding of what it's like to be her and ways we are alike. I'm filled with love and admiration as we walk side by side. Then we spiral apart, and the chasm opens back up.

◯

As a young woman, my mother briefly went to college, the only one in her family to do so. "I had saved enough money for two years," she tells me at dinner one evening; "but my older brother had a new 'invention'; he was always full of schemes. He asked to borrow money from me. He was sure it would make him rich and then he would pay me back. I didn't want to give it to him, but my mother told me I should. He didn't get rich, and he didn't pay me back. I had to leave school after one year."

I'm crushed for her, seventy-five years later. When the US, and her beloved, entered World War II, she moved back and forth across the country. From Tennessee, where she met my father, she traveled by train to Washington State—sight unseen—to work for the war effort as a secretary at Spokane's Geiger Field Air Force Base. When my father finished meteorology training in New York City and was stationed in Dallas, she moved to Texas to marry him. He deployed to Europe six weeks later, and she moved to Michigan to live with his parents for a year, and then to Florida to live with hers. With each move she changed civil service jobs, taking care of herself and writing to her new husband every other day.

She lost her fierce independence after my father returned from Europe, or at least buried it. It wasn't the era of independent wives. Married women quit their jobs and returned to the kitchen. I suppose that was my mother's dream all along. It was mine as well when I finished college, until my life took the unexpected divorce turn, and then I wasn't prepared to support myself. I returned to school at age forty for a graduate degree in school counseling, taking a play from my mother's example: changing course when life called for it. I found an independence that I couldn't seem to grasp while I was partnered.

In the seventeen years since my father died—after fifty-one years of marriage—Mama rediscovered her autonomy as I had. She found people to do the work around the property my father had once taken care of: preparing beds for gardening, mowing the lawn and meadow, cleaning debris from the flat roof (or doing it herself), getting the garbage to the dump, making house repairs, and doing routine maintenance. She found plumbers and furnace technicians, tree-removers and electricians, and she supervised them all. She doggedly dealt with the finances, even if not the way her husband or daughters would have.

Though her mind seems sharp, at least to the casual listener, she is losing her sight, her hearing, and her memory at a frightening pace. She probably has always suffered from undiagnosed depression. Many days she spirals deeper into the murk, adapting to her changing physical state, if not with grace. She walks with a cane outside now—upgrading from her broomstick in the months since my arrival—and holds onto walls and furniture inside; she stands in front of the kitchen counter with feet spread wide for stability. The fear of falling and breaking brittle bones is constantly with her. She must be careful and thoughtful of every morsel of food she puts in her mouth lest her bowel becomes obstructed and lands her in pain in the hospital for treatment that will not include surgery, the only solution that might have helped when she was younger. She is obsessed with the movement of her bowels to give her a signal that she is okay for another day. Her partner in life is long gone. Friends are dead, lost in a minefield of memory loss, or have moved away to live closer to children. That she still gets up every morning in the face of all the loss is extraordinary to me.

One by one, my sisters and I infiltrate the arenas of her life, robbing her of decision-making, because it is necessary. As everything she cannot control—in spite of her valiant attempts—continues in free fall, she clings to control of what she can, or thinks she can; things that seem inconsequential to me, but are of enormous import to her. She resists most of our suggestions to make her life easier or safer. I go about picking up the traces of her life, trying to fit them together into a sense-making whole without her knowing it. Of course that is impossible, and both of us are left with chaos and frustration.

Apparently, I have a colossal need for control too. I fight her idiosyncrasies as if my sanity depends on it, but her control of what she can still control is her weapon against the loss of everything else. If she needs all the blinds closed at night, we will close the blinds every night.

"Why?" I ask, curious.

"To keep the bugs from being attracted to the light from the lamp and smashing into the windows," she says. When I ask why not just turn the light off at night, she tells me she leaves it on so prowlers will know we are home. None of that makes sense to me, but I let it go. It's how she has always done it, it's what has made her feel safe living here alone in a big house with many doors and windows, beyond the vision of neighbors. In accepting her need for control, I must give up mine. Or try to.

◆

When disaster strikes again, Rebecca and I take the next big step toward assuming the reins.

14

November

Expanding the Care Circle

Mama reached overhead to put a vase in a cupboard above the dryer and strained her back. Rebecca and I have both been on duty ever since—she closing her store or paying someone to be there. We struggle to manage our irritation with Mama's creaky, high-pitched whining and exaggerated moaning. Nothing we do to try to alleviate her pain or make her more comfortable is right.

We are both at the house around the clock, except for grocery and drugstore runs that give one of us at a time a break. I rejoice when a train blocks the crossing between the foot of the hill and town and adds five minutes to my time away.

It takes both of us to get her to the bathroom. When the extra strength Tylenol isn't touching the pain, and Rebecca goes down the hill to get Tylenol with codeine—a prescription saved from her last hospital visit—I have to get her out of bed and to the toilet on my own.

"Hold onto my arm with both hands," I tell her. "Let me pull you up."

In the way of the minister performing a baptism at the Baptist church I attended and was employed by in Raleigh, I position her hands in opposite directions on my right forearm, and slip my left arm under her shoulders, relatively painlessly raising her to sitting.

"How did you know to do that?" she asks. I can't tell if she's impressed or merely curious.

"Years of watching immersion baptisms," I tell her, pleased that something at least has worked, after failing again at my "breathe through the pain" Lamaze lesson. Though my church was a progressive American Baptist affiliate, I wonder if my words take her back to her Southern Baptist days before her decades as a Presbyterian and, following my father's death, a Methodist, with their sprinkle baptisms.

The next time she can't remember to let me do the lifting, and no amount of instruction is helpful.

◡

Three days later Mama has improved enough for Rebecca to return to work. *Surrender* becomes my word as I carry the monitor receiver around the house with me during the day, often hanging out on the living room sofa waiting for Mama—who's still bedridden—to need something. My laptop is my lifeline, and the familiar voices of NPR and encouragement from friends via email form a narrow band beyond my confinement. Facebook is my guilty pleasure as I stalk the lives of acquaintances I never kept up with before, and silently rage at friends who don't "do" Facebook, leaving me feeling estranged. This is what it's like to be a true caregiver. It's full-time work being at someone's beck and call, and not much else gets done. I long to call my Raleigh circle of friends and invite them to the house for dinner. I have yet to make any local friends, and for the first time, I'm lonely.

When Mama finally falls asleep, and I close my eyes for a nap myself, the landline phone—the ringer set heart-attack loud—pierces the silence in the dining room a few feet from my chair and on the extension phone that rests on my father's side of Mama's bed. It's like finally getting a restless toddler down for a nap, and a Jehovah's Witness rings the doorbell and wakes the baby.

"I didn't sign up for this," I text-whine to a friend as I hear Mama talking on the phone.

"You kind of did," he says.

I guess he's right. What was I thinking? Tylenol with codeine is working for Mama's pain—when I can talk her into taking it—and I'm having wine for mine.

❧

It's a wake-up call. I can't sustain this kind of caregiving alone, and we had best get our ducks in a row before the next crisis. Should we move her or get care for her at home? We have no idea which she would prefer.

Rebecca hears from a customer about a geriatric social worker in Olympia who might be able to help us assess needs and offer solutions. I call him and, with Mama's skeptical acquiescence, he comes to the house one morning.

David is a small man about my age with a greying beard and small bright eyes behind round-framed glasses. He has worked for nearly forty years with people with many flavors of dementia and with their families and caregivers. Rebecca and I sit at the dining room table with Mama. Jo Ann joins us via FaceTime on my laptop at the head of the table in what was our father's customary dinner place. Unlike Rebecca and me, who look more like Mama, Jo Ann is all our father, with her auburn hair—from a bottle now—ruddy complexion, and the aquiline nose of our paternal grandmother. I wish he were at the table. I wish he hadn't refused to move to a retirement community with Mama years ago, as she wanted, so she could have started a new life with him by her side. I'm angry with him now for his selfishness.

David seems to understand immediately and compassionately what we are dealing with. He makes continuous eye contact as he talks with Mama, his head bobbing encouragingly with each point he makes.

"What are you enjoying about your life?" he asks her.

She's quiet for a long moment, thinking.

"I like to walk on the deck," she says finally, "but I have to close my eyes if the sun is bright."

"So you feel safe walking on the deck even with your eyes closed," he says, mirroring her words, his head nodding.

Brilliant, I think. It's a technique I know about from school counseling days, but haven't thought to use with Mama.

"Yes," she says.

"And you would miss that if you couldn't live here." It's an affirmation, not a question.

"I would. In the house I know where all the furniture is and I can use it and the wall to get around."

"Even though your vision is fading, you can 'see' here, because it's familiar. Do you use a cane?" he asks.

"Not in the house," she says quickly, with what sounds like pride.

"What else do you enjoy?" David asks, bobbing, his eyes growing wide behind his glasses.

"I enjoy making my breakfast, and eating by myself," she says. "I like time alone. Gretchen cooks dinner; I can't see to do that anymore. But I can't always eat what she cooks."

Rebecca and I exchange a glance. David ignores the rider.

He continues to lead her through what it's like for her at home, then helps her explore what it might be like to live at the residential facility.

"I couldn't get around by myself," she admits. "And I couldn't eat the food. I can't hear in groups of people." She's quiet then while David waits, but she says nothing more. She looks far away.

"It sounds like you are doing well here. Would you like to keep living at home?" he asks then, his eyebrows lifted, questioning.

"I should have moved a long time ago," she says. She pauses. "But maybe I wouldn't still be alive if I had left."

"Would you like to move now?" he asks.

She's quiet again. "I guess I should," she says.

He leans closer. "Would you rather stay here, if you could choose?" I don't feel he is leading the witness, but trying to get her to dig deep. I need to know what she wants.

"I don't want to ruin my daughters' lives," she says.

"I think they want what is best for you," David says, "but they would like to know what you want for yourself right now."

Tears form in her eyes. "I would like to stay here as long as I can," she says quietly. "Is that okay?" she asks, looking at me and Rebecca.

"Yes," we both say.

Her tears fall freely then. "I'm so fortunate!" she says, weeping. "I never thought I would be able to stay in my home."

Oh my God, what just happened? I lose track of the conversation. *I only meant to get her to live in the moment and be happy to stay until I'm ready to go. And now I will feel guilty moving her ever, knowing she doesn't want to go.*

Don't look too far ahead, I hear an old friend whispering in my ear. *If you don't have a plan for your life, someone else does* niggles in my other ear. Rebecca promised not to let me get stuck. I have a feeling the pinky swear was far short of a contract; we should have pricked fingers. Panic bubbles up as I flash on my future. I'm going to be sick.

I jerk my attention back to the table.

"I suggest you find a caregiver for several hours a week to help keep Gretchen from burning out," David is saying, addressing Mama directly. "It will happen quickly. Caring for a parent is hard work!"

Someone understands. I nearly weep with relief. Mama should understand too, she cared for her mother, who was challenging. But all she remembers is her perception, in retrospect, that she let her mother down. She is silent. She looks like I feel, shell-shocked, and I wonder if she feels I have let her down.

"There's a small agency in Chehalis," he tells us. "I think they could find help for you. How does that sound, Stellajoe?"

Mama is quiet for so long, her head bowed, I think she's gone to sleep. "Okay," she says finally, stunning me with non-argumentative consent.

David looks up the contact information for me and I walk him to the door.

"She was on her best behavior," I tell him, "articulate and rational." I'm a little disappointed that she hasn't shown her true nature, but I needn't be.

"I know," he assures me. "And, believe me, I know this is hard work. Would you like to meet with me privately at my office? I can give you some coping strategies, and information on how dementia is affecting her."

"Yes. Thank you." I burst into pent up tears. He's thrown me a lifeline, and I grab on.

∼

The hunt begins for a caregiver, all the while Mama insisting she doesn't need one. I realize now she agreed to it because she wanted David to go away; she didn't want to talk about it anymore.

"I'm sorry," I say, "I know it isn't what you want. But, if I'm going to stay with you, we have to hire regular help."

"You don't have to stay here, Gretchen," she says. "I can sell the house and move to Colonial." I breathe in through my nose, out through my mouth, in and out.

The last time she pulled moving to the Residence out of her bag, my sisters were ready to call her bluff and say, "Let's go." I argued against it since her irrational insistence that she will have to sell the house to move there would leave me homeless—failing to consider the months it would take to clean out the house even to get it on the market. I promised her a year; did she promise me a year too? We should have talked details.

We know it won't be easy to have a regular employee. Mama is accustomed to telling her helpers in the past—currently Michelle, whom she's known since Michelle was a child, and Stan the Handy Man, who is a man, handy to have around to do jobs Mama considers men's work—to come when she asks for them. When she wants to be alone or doesn't have anything for them to do, they comply when she tells them not to come at the last minute, as if they come as a favor to her, not because they are trying to earn a living. Since my arrival, Michelle, a professional caregiver with regular clients, has rarely come.

Michelle, a pretty woman, slender and blond, a few years younger than I am, quietly does whatever Mama asks of her and, unlike me, patiently accepts corrective instruction. She is an obsessive-compulsive cleaner while I only do minimal post-dinner kitchen cleanup, leaving the rest to Stan and Michelle. I have never since childhood met Mama's stringent cleaning standards, and I'm not stepping into that sinkhole again. Now we are asking Mama to adapt to the scheduled presence of someone else in the house, along with me, which is bad enough. She will have to train them in her ways and, I fear, will never be satisfied with their performance. I fervently wish Michelle were available mornings. She has set a high bar.

~

I quickly hire Jill for two mornings a week through the agency David recommended, and congratulate myself in the great luck at getting her. For one thing, having cared for her father until his death, she understands *my* need. "It's harder to care for your own parent than it is for someone else's," she reassures me. Two mornings a week doesn't meet the agency's minimum time requirement, but they agree to it with the expectation that the hours will increase.

I feel newfound peace the first week, doing my own thing during the mornings Jill is here, knowing Mama is occupied. Mama isn't willing to give up Michelle, though, who agrees to keep coming on the usual sporadic schedule, a fiasco waiting to happen.

~

Two weeks after we hire Jill, Mama tells me she told Jill not to come the next morning.

"You can't do that!" I say. I take a breath and calm myself. "We have a contract with Jill. If you tell her not to come, we have to pay her anyway."

"It's my life, Gretchen," she says, "and I make my own decisions."

"We made this one as a family," I say gently. "You can't just change it without a discussion."

She sighs. "*You* call her then and tell her to come."

The next morning, Mama calls me at the coffee shop at nine twenty.

"Jill isn't here yet. Did you call her and tell her to come?"

"Yes," I tell her for the third time. "I'm sure she will be there, but it isn't time yet."

"I thought she comes at nine o'clock."

"No, she comes at nine thirty."

"Okaaaay," she says in her you-don't-know-what-you're-talking-about voice.

When I return home at noon with groceries, Jill is leaving, dismissed thirty minutes ahead of schedule. She's kind about it; I'm furious. I know it's because Mama arranged for Michelle to come, choosing to fix the overlap after I pointed it out by trying to cancel Jill, then by sending her home early. She doesn't like two people in the house at the same time—it's "confusing"—or even the same day—"it's tiring." Yet she insists on scheduling them herself and can't remember when she has told them to come.

"Your mom thought I was late and wasn't coming," Jill says with a smile.

I close my eyes and sigh.

"I reminded her of the hours we agreed on, and that I would add Fridays in December. She said she didn't need me on Fridays, that you think she needs help more than she does. I quit another job so I could make you my priority. I don't know what to do."

I take a deep breath and expel it. I don't know what to do either. "I'm sorry," I tell her. "I'll talk to her. Messing with your hours is not acceptable."

"This is really hard," she says, putting her hand on my shoulder.

"I know."

◞◞

My stomach is in a knot all afternoon, anticipating the confrontation to come.

Mama gets up from her nap—taken too late because Michelle was here—while I'm cooking dinner. I decide not to address the additional hours and focus on the current schedule.

"Mama," I say, "you can't shorten Jill's schedule at the last minute. This is how she earns her living. What can I do to help you?"

Mama's face clouds. "I don't know what you're talking about."

Ignoring her denial I say, "Would it be easier for you if I take charge of the scheduling to make sure your helpers don't come on the same days?"

"If I can't schedule the people I'm paying," she snaps, "then I won't have the help."

I back off. One battle at a time. For now I just need to get her to accept Jill.

After Rebecca and I talk it over—realizing we should have interviewed several people and included Mama in the process—we persuade her to stick with Jill until the end of the year and promise we will reevaluate then. I didn't know getting help would be such hard work.

15

November

Dementia Education

The winter rains have set in with zeal. It's grey. Mama, who has always slumped in fall and winter, is grey too, and more irritable than ever. She digs in her heels in opposition to Jill each time the smallest thing is unsatisfactory. Jill, a small woman about my age with short sandy curls, meets many of Mama's criteria—or one at least: she's a small, quiet presence. But she isn't Michelle, and Mama can't adjust.

"Jill can't read a recipe." "I can't understand her voice." "She talks too loud." "She doesn't talk loud enough." "She's not clean in the kitchen." "Her car isn't comfortable." "She does things I didn't ask her to do." *I don't want to need help.*

One rare sunny day when Jill is at the house in the morning and Stan is coming in the afternoon, I take off for the mountains. I don't get very far up a forest service road when snow stops me. It's okay. I got out of the house to someplace I could breathe. I pull off the road and walk through the snow for a ways, then drive back to the small town of Randle and sit in the car and eat my lunch and read. I must not lose these escapes or I won't survive this time. I should be considering what I want next in my life, but I can't visualize a "next."

❧

Following the debacle with Jill's schedule, I make my first appointment with David. We meet in the conference room at the memory care facility in Olympia where he consults with clients and families. He tells me his objective is to make sure I am taking care of myself, to be a resource for me to vent and ask questions, to validate that what I am doing is emotionally and psychologically hard. And to give me information about what is happening in my mother's brain. I wonder if the day will come that she will be living in this facility—or that I will be.

"She doesn't want a regular caregiver," I tell him when he asks how it's going. "She's fighting it like crazy."

"The truth is," he tells me, "she is beyond the ability to make a decision. The rub is she doesn't realize that. You have to make decisions for her. And she is going to resist with all she has."

"She says things that aren't true, and insists she is right and I am wrong. Like about the hours we hired Jill for."

"The big picture is this," he says, his eyebrows rising and his head nodding, punctuating his point, "the facts no longer matter. At ninety-six, with diminishing short-term memory and brain function, your mother is no longer bound to the facts. Nothing, including words, is where it's supposed to be. Her frustration level is very high. She has a low threshold of tolerance for the pieces she knows are missing and for being challenged with the truth. Conversation is no longer an exchange of information; what matters now are feelings."

"But she's not a feelings person," I argue. "She loves information, and it makes her a little bit crazy when I don't know—or care about—details. And how can I let go of *my* need for her facts to be correct?"

"It's okay when she gets the facts all wrong," David says. "Don't try to straighten it out. Look to what she is trying to do: stay in control. Learn to discern when reality matters, which is rarely, and when to play along. Figure out what she wants to hear and give it to her. Agreeing with her version of reality will make her feel safe and secure."

I sigh. This goes against everything I have known her to be. But then, maybe I didn't know her. Now, staying in control is her everything, and it doesn't matter who she takes down to achieve it. That's all I need to know.

David is gentle and kind, and he accepts without judgment my frustration and my remorse that I can't do this better. I know already I will depend on him to be a place I can vent and cry, even as I struggle to understand that, contrary to how it seems, my mother is not "business as usual." Her brain is failing.

"It's confabulation," he goes on, seeing my frustration, "and we all do it. We tell our stories and fill in the gaps. Our own stories are pretty good; it's hard for the uninitiated to see where reality meets fiction. The fault lines are bigger with dementia, sometimes enormous. In the elderly, reality is the smaller piece. The task of convincing themselves that they are capable is their primary job. They want desperately to keep it together, and they are terrified. So what they don't know for sure, they make up. Then they convince themselves that it's true, and stick to the story—until they change it."

I struggle to wrap my brain around this information. In Mama's case, the difference between reality and confabulation seems more subtle than in the case of those with Alzheimer's-type dementia. Mama sounds so reasonable and so sure of herself, and sometimes she's right when I think she's wrong.

"It seems not to be forgetfulness, but intentional invention of fact to suit her desire," I tell David.

"But, actually, it is forgetfulness," he says again, "and so the invention of fact."

Just as she refuses to give up on her body by believing what she eats or another doctor or more exercise or refusing to nap will save her, I can't give up on her mind. But it only frustrates her when I challenge her irrationality and contradictions. It's a cosmic dance in which I will forget and remember, forget and remember her reality. I'm in denial too.

But I can free her from being bound to facts, tell her what she wants to hear, and respond in ways that will increase her sense of well-being. Letting her be in control of her reality is the gift I can give. Perhaps letting go of my own need to be right will be a gift I can give to myself.

I am under no illusion it will be easy, but understanding a bit better why she is so maddening is a big step forward. Getting this one thing right will become my work. I will fail again and again, and never give up trying.

∾

David's bill for his time with all of us, along with my hour at his office, comes to the house. Mama wants to know what the additional charge is. I had hoped not to tell her; I consider it therapy, and therefore confidential. I am also expecting her to pay for it. It's a dilemma.

"I met with him privately," I tell her.

"What did he say?"

"He helped me understand how things are for you and how I might respond helpfully rather than antagonistically." That seems to satisfy her, and I let out the breath I didn't realize I was holding. I feel like I've been caught being unfaithful.

When she sends the check to David I can see through the sealed envelope she has included a note. When she pays a bill herself, she doesn't seal the envelope so I can make sure the check has been written correctly. I carefully open it and read: *The charges were not made clear to me and I will accept no further charges unless I know about them ahead of time.*

If I want his support, I have to tell her I am seeing him and get her permission.

16

December

Retreat

My old new town sits in a valley in a county that, though narrow from north to south, extends east and west nearly from the mountains to the sea. It's a maze of farmland valleys and evergreen-covered hills. In late summer and early fall, when the morning fog gave way to glorious blue skies, I jumped in the car and took off for the mountains or an exploration of the valleys of Lewis County, grateful when Mama was able to fend for herself. Now, in the dark damp days of winter, opportunities for the adventures that are critical to my self-care are rare. As Mama sinks deeper into her winter low, it's hard to be away, even with a part-time caregiver.

One bright day, though, I take a solo car venture to the southern end of the Washington coast, leaving Rebecca on call and giving Mama some solitude. In an attempt to share my life, I tell her my plan to have lunch at the historic hotel near Willapa Bay.

"Well," she says, "it might take you longer than you expect."

"I have no expectations," I say calmly. She will not deny me pleasure.

"It will take longer if the roads are slick."

"Yep," I say, breathing.

"It's a two-lane road; you will have to go slower."

"I know it's two lanes. It's why I'm going there."

"There's probably a lot of logging traffic on that road during the week."

"It's Sunday." I kiss her cheek and say goodbye.

∽

It's a beautiful day. The sun sparkles on the frosty fields and barn roofs. Hoar frost lines the edges of the red and green salal and Oregon grape along the road, and trickles of water coming out of rock outcroppings are tiny frozen waterfalls. When I spot a pair of swans swimming among the reeds in the shallows of the bay, I pull off the road and watch them play for a while. Later I sit beside a blazing fire in the inn's fireplace to eat my lunch and read.

On the way home, I stop to drive through Washington's only in-use covered bridge that Mama learned about from her current recorded book so I can tell her I saw it when she asks, as I know she will. She is coming to enjoy living my adventures vicariously, one of our few points of connection. She was an adventurer too, hiking in the Appalachian Mountains with friends as a young woman, honeymooning in the Rockies, camping with her husband and children in the Pacific Northwest, driving the county backroads with my father after we children left home, walking in the woods beside our house. I am her adventures now, my deep-soul passion springing directly from her.

∽

Last month, in an uncharacteristic financial splurge, I registered for a weeklong writing retreat on Whidbey Island after Thanksgiving. With Mama's agreement, I arranged for Michelle to spend the nights

I would be away so Rebecca didn't have to during her busy retail season.

The night before I leave, I'm as excited as a child on Christmas Eve. As we finish eating dinner—the last I'll have to cook for a week—Mama tells me she doesn't need Michelle to spend the night while I'm gone.

"Perhaps not," I say, "but Rebecca and I can't do what we need to do if we are worrying about you alone at night."

"I can press my Lifeline button and they'll call Rebecca and 911."

"That's a good back up," I say, trying not to explode in frustration, "but it just doesn't feel like the best solution."

She gets to what she's really feeling then, and my heart breaks for her.

"I miss time alone."

"I understand that so well," I say, gently then, knowing what it took for her to pull it from her depths. "But Michelle will only be here at night. Jill will be here on Wednesday morning. Other than that you will be alone every day until the weekend when Rebecca comes."

At that moment Michelle calls to say hello and tells Mama she is looking forward to being here. It is exactly what Mama needed, and I don't hear any more about it.

◠

I arrive early at Aldermarsh Retreat Center in my excitement to leave home, and nab one of the two tiny rustic cottages, as opposed to a bedroom in one of the houses. I am so happy I can hardly breathe. With no running water, Spirit House has a pee pot, a ceramic wash basin and a pitcher of water, an electric tea kettle. There's a double bed in the alcove with three low windows around its head, through which I will hear the coyotes and owls. A ladder leads to the loft where I will write in the treetops under the two skylights.

There is no internet connection in my cottage, and I can't get cell service on the grounds. I walk up to the road and get two bars. Enough to send Rebecca a text saying I got here and won't be calling. She writes back that Mama said she didn't know until this morning that someone would be with her every night. I breathe it away into the treetops.

17

December

Abbott and Costello

I return home rested and full. There is no happy homecoming.

"I won't be having Jill here three days a week," Mama says over salmon, mashed potatoes, and spinach.

I continue eating in silence, waiting to see where this is going.

"She makes me tired. All I can do while she's in the house is go to bed or sit in the chair." Perhaps she is remembering long gone days when that wasn't what she did anyway. Or when there was no one around to witness it.

"Maybe if you want to be more active, Jill could do some things with you that you aren't able to do by yourself," I say brightly. "You have been saying you want to be able to go visit people; Jill could take you!"

"I don't have the energy for that," she says; "I want them to come here."

"Then you will have to invite them. Jill can help you get ready to entertain them."

"I wish you wouldn't bring up caregivers while I'm eating, Gretchen. It upsets my stomach."

She brought it up, but I keep quiet. She misses her solitude. I'm the one who has shattered it, and she can't send me away.

We both want our old lives back.

❧

I persuade Mama to add Fridays to Jill's schedule in December, as agreed, but by the middle of the month she is messing with the schedule so much that Jill has no idea what to do about the client opportunities she continues to turn down. It's time to talk—again. For once, I remember to ask Mama when would be a good time. She chooses today, before dinner. It's a conversation to rival Abbott and Costello's "Who's on First?"

At the dining room table, she with her back to the window and I looking out through the fir branches toward the valley, praying the tranquil view will guide me, I ask her what she wants Jill's schedule to be for the rest of the month.

"It's not what I want, it's what I need," she says.

"Okay, what do you need?" I say.

"I think I need to call Colonial Residence and see if they have a place available similar to the one I turned down before. If they do, I need to take it."

"Well, that is a conversation we can have some time. But it's not going to happen before Christmas. So when would you like Jill to come the rest of the month?"

"Well, I told her I don't need her three days a week."

"Okay, when do you want her?"

"Was she here yesterday?"

"Yes."

"I only want her twice a week."

"And what two days do you want her?"

"I only want her twice a week," she repeats.

"And when do you want her?"

She slides down the rabbit hole of getting someone "more suit-able," who doesn't talk so loud, who has a car that's comfortable, who doesn't use a paper towel to wipe a spill from the floor when she knows there are rags. I let her talk, countering her complaints only a couple of times.

"I don't think make and model of their car is a criteria for a care-giver; the next one might drive a pickup," I say. Michelle and Jill have the same make and model of car, but I don't ask why one is comfort-able and one is not.

"I think I just need to move to Colonial Residence."

"And then you wouldn't get to go anywhere," I say, teetering at the edge of the hole.

"Michelle said she would come and get me and take me places. When she can."

We sit in silence for a moment. Her face wistful, me sad for her.

"Maybe it's just that I want to be able to do it myself. And I know that I can't."

"That is very perceptive," I say gently. "I wish you could still do it yourself too. Let's talk about the rest of this month." Realizing we need to take it day-by-day, I break it down. "Did you tell Jill to come tomorrow?"

"I thought we were talking about next week."

"First this week. When do you want her? Tomorrow?"

"Yes, I think I told her to come tomorrow."

"Okay, so you don't want her on Friday?"

"Yes, she can come on Friday."

"And next week when do you want her?"

"Do I have to know now?"

"Yes. This is her livelihood, and she turned down a job last week because she was scheduled here, and then she was sent home early and she could have taken the job. And that isn't fair."

"I didn't know that."

"Do you want her Monday?"

"Yes."

"And what other day?"

"Well, the same as this week."

"So, Monday, Wednesday, and Friday?"

"Yes."

It takes fifty minutes to determine that we are sticking with the original schedule, albeit with shorter hours, a compromise. And I keep my cool through the entire conversation. I pour myself a victory glass of wine while I finish preparing dinner.

The next day, Mama sweetly reports to Jill the change in hours, adding, "If you get more hours somewhere else, don't hesitate to take the job." Jill immediately accepts a request for more hours from one of her other clients, and we will have to release her at the end of the month. Mama seems pleased. I'm ready to throw myself from a moving train.

∽

A week later, Michelle tells Mama she has hurt her back and can't come her two hours a week for at least the next month. Providing for all Mama's needs is back in my lap.

The lesson we have learned is to include Mama in decisions every step of the way. Her verbal agreement is not the same as buy-in, and she is not going to let us run over her. Maybe we should have vetted several people, but it wouldn't have made any difference. She doesn't want to need anyone but me, and she pretends she doesn't need me either.

I have a fantasy of eating tomato soup and a grilled cheese sandwich in front of a fire while watching some insipid Christmas movie with Smudge in my lap. I want it so viscerally I sink to the floor in the corner of the kitchen and weep. And then I cook fish, chard, and acorn squash, with a side of canned peaches for Mama, and sit at the table for an hour, knitting fingerless mittens and looking out the window into the early winter darkness until she is done.

"Does your mother live with you?" people ask when they hear I am a family caregiver. That she has joined my household and adjusted herself to my life is the expectation. What self-respecting, healthy, active, attractive sixty-year-old lives with her mother? Jane Gross writes, "If Mom lives with you, you've won best-in-show among daughters. AARP calls you the backbone of the nation's long-term care system." In a massive assumption, Gross adds, "You'd better have a saintly husband." None of the helpful books I read address children who live in their parent's home, because who does that? It is surely a special hell.

∿

I'm not sure I'm making Mama's life any better, and I'm afraid my friends will forget me. I'm afraid *I* will forget me. A friend reminds me in a text from Raleigh, "This is not your forever." I'm not so sure. There are 210 days left of my original commitment, but now I don't know if there is an end. I'm missing the countdown.

18

January

Anger Management

I sleepwalk through Christmas, missing my children, who, with their spouses and Max and Ethan, joined their dad and large stepfamily for Christmas on the East Coast. When their father and I divorced, I idealistically hoped we could navigate our "family apart" nontraditionally, perhaps even doing holidays together, rather than be a house divided. But while our families are cordial, my vision was never embraced by anyone else. As long as their dad and I lived in the same town, we each had holiday time with our children. Now I'm far away, and it's the first Christmas in thirty-three years I haven't seen them. I am awash with envy of their big fun family time with Gens Y and Z.

Jo Ann and her husband, Peter, come from Virginia, and their children from Seattle drive down for Christmas day. I'm still in charge of everything, having to ask for help and wishing they would just take over. Their presence does nothing to assuage my longing for my family.

When Peter goes home to return to work, leaving only Jo Ann in the house with me and Mama, I'm wrung out and without ambition. I can't do anything right. I overhear or am sympathetically told all Mama tells Jo Ann I am doing wrong and Jo Ann's responding defense of me.

"Gretchen likes her routines; I am more flexible," I hear Mama say, referring to my fierce hold on the weekly coffee shop and writing time that has been my practice for more than a decade. It's ironic, coming from the Queen of Habit, and I hear Jo Ann smothering laughter.

As we eat the dinner I prepared for New Years' Eve, Mama speaks up. "Michelle says she might be able to come late afternoons in a couple of weeks, if her back is feeling better."

"That's nice," I say, "but it's when you nap." Michelle previously spent most of her time with Mama in the kitchen, which is where I need to be, preparing dinner, in late afternoon. I also don't want precious caregiver hours squandered at a time of day I can't leave the house, but I don't say so.

As if she has heard my inner thought, Mama says, "Well, maybe she can cook my dinner." My breath leaves my body.

"Is my cooking not satisfactory?" I ask when I recover. Though she complains all the time, I didn't think it would come to this. I refrain from reminding her of Michelle's inability to make hot cereal, soup, and chocolate chip cookies to Mama's specifications.

"I can't always eat what you cook, and sometimes it's dry. You don't tell me what you are planning, and I don't know until that day what I think I can eat. And I don't like the way you thaw meat. You need to take it out of the freezer the night before and let it thaw in the refrigerator. It dries out when you 'quick-thaw' it in the microwave."

"How can I take meat out of the freezer the night before if you don't know until midafternoon what you feel like eating that night?" She says nothing. I know she's trying to stay in untenable control of her living, that that's what all her complaints are about. I'm learning not to push her, but this time I want to know what's in her head.

"Are you going to answer me?" I ask, admirably containing my rising ire.

"No," she says.

I sigh and let it go. *You are not a fuck up,* I whisper to myself. *She is old.*

∾

"Gretchen!" Mama's voice reaches me in the living room where I'm relaxing after dinner while she cleans up in the kitchen. I blow out air as my head flops back against the sofa cushion. I wish I could call out a response, but she wouldn't hear me.

"What do you need?" I ask, entering the kitchen, wondering why the hell Jo Ann isn't in here.

"You put the forks in the wrong place in the dishwasher rack and I stabbed myself when I emptied it because I can't see."

I follow the Rule of the Forks religiously, but she did not tell the house guests where to put them, and now it's all on me. In pent up frustration, hurt, and depletion, I'm an explosion waiting for a match, and she struck it. My admirable control vaporizes.

"I always put the forks in the right place! I'm not the only one loading the dishwasher!" My voice gets louder and higher as I throw in the kitchen sink: "And why, when someone takes you to the store, do you buy brands you tell me not to get? I go to three grocery stores so I can get what you want! Is it not really necessary?" *Stop!* my head screams.

"They don't have the right brand of spinach at Fullers," she says calmly, seemingly deliberately countering my raised voice.

"I know that," I rage on, ignoring my inner voice, "it's why I get it at Safeway, so why did you get the Fuller's brand? And we had two bags of spinach anyway!"

She is tough, but my wrath is too much this time. She falls apart.

Bent double, heaving and sobbing, she staggers down the hall to her bed, holding onto the wall to keep her balance. I put myself in time out in my bedroom.

Later Jo Ann tells me she was moaning over and over that she hates herself and she shouldn't be alive. Neither should I. What is the matter with me that I scream at an old woman who is doing the best she can?

When she returns to herself, Mama tells Jo Ann I need anger management counseling. I do have a short fuse, like my father did, rare but explosive, and quickly dissipated, and lately not that rare. My ability to get it out and then gone is a childhood quality Mama used to tell me she loved about me. If there is anything she loves about me now, she is unable to give it words. *It's cognitive dysfunction,* I remind myself. It doesn't help.

Jo Ann tells her I handle anger very well, setting it free rather than bottling it up. "And she has a therapist," she adds, asking if she would pay for me to continue to see David, and understand it's confidential and not to ask about it. When she relates the conversation to me, she tells me Mama agreed to the proposal, but Mama says nothing to me.

Maybe every primary caregiver should have a distant sibling who can do no wrong. In spite of my frustration—and envy—that Jo Ann can orbit from afar while I am stuck in the nucleus, I'm grateful for her intercessory contribution, and irritated that she never picks up the phone and offers it long distance.

❧

I immediately send David an email for an appointment and meet with him in his Olympia office two days later.

"She has so many food issues," I tell him, "and they aren't all about irritable bowel syndrome. I have to buy certain brands at certain stores and she checks the 'buy by' dates, and I can't buy fresh vegetables out of season, and I have to thaw meat according to her specifications, and what she liked one day she doesn't like on another, and what she couldn't eat yesterday she wants today, and she complains about how I cook *everything.* I'm so tired."

David waits for me to get it all out, nodding his head compassionately. I begin to cry as I relate the spinach story.

"I hate that I upset her. But I really wanted to know why she and Jo Ann bought the brand she tells me not to buy. Why does she make my life insane and doesn't want to put anyone else out? Why wouldn't she answer me?" I'm sobbing now.

Gently he says, "This is the kind of question she is incapable of answering. She doesn't see the flaw in her reasoning, and pointing it out to her confuses her to the point of communication shut down. The brains of those in cognitive decline can't compute facts."

It's a fact I can't seem to remember.

"Your job is to let her get facts wrong."

"So I have to let her tell me *I* am wrong? I don't think I can do it."

"This is really hard work," he reminds me.

Knowledge is power, I tell myself as I drive home. I do not feel powerful.

❧

With my sisters' approval, David sets up a PayPal account, and I put the expense on Mama's credit card where it gets lost in the ocean of all she can no longer see to examine. She doesn't have to know when I see him. I feel like the unscrupulous child embezzling funds from the unaware parent. When does it stop being the Therapeutic Lie and start being unethical? I only know that if I am to survive this, I need to use all the resources available to me.

19

January

Courage

Though Mama agreed to a grab bar on the side of the tub and a stool in back in case she needs it, she fiercely defends her ability to shower herself. I feel it's no longer safe for her to be unattended. We find a compromise. I wait in her bedroom, watching through a tiny opening in the pocket door between her room and the bathroom to be sure she's in and out okay. When she gets out of the shower, she sits on the toilet seat to dry herself and then calls me to put lotion on her back.

I rub the lotion down her twisted spine, ravaged by scoliosis, moving around the curves and over the knobs, my hands like skis on a mogul trail. Her once five feet four inches has shrunken as her backbone permanently bends forward and sideward. Her paper-thin skin is stretched tight, as if it can barely hold her brittle skeleton together.

Her skin is well beyond the changing terrain of my own aging skin. I have freckles that never used to be there and white, pigment-free spots, but hers is a canvas of color. Her torso is dotted with tiny red blood dots—harmless "cherry angiomas," I read on WebMD. Ever-present bruises in shades of purple and green paint her hands, wrists, and shins where she knocks against furniture and corners. Red and blue veins and arteries, clearly visible beneath the surface of her skin, rope through her arms and legs, the backs of her hands, the tops of her feet—a topographical road map of the highways on which she has traveled through life for nearly a century.

She makes an annual visit to the dermatologist to have the crusty, precancerous carcinomas—perhaps the result of growing up in the sunny South—frozen into submission. The last time I took her, I quietly told the doctor we didn't want to treat the one that tested positive, and asked him not to tell her about it. It won't be what puts her in the earth.

The skin of her face is soft and wrinkled and hangs loosely; her milky blue eyes gaze quietly out beneath the ever-present visor that shades the permanently dilated left eye, the one that still has a gradually fading pinpoint of vision. "You will never be blind," her glaucoma doctor told her, rather impatiently. I took him at his word. Mama didn't believe it for a minute.

Her ears are out of proportion, now, to her wizened head; one holds a hearing aid, the other long silenced. The lustrous strawberry-blond hair her future husband was smitten by when they were courting is whiter than white and too thin to hide her pink scalp. "Is my coat covered with hairs?" she asks me when we go out. I'm already beginning to find my own white hair in places other than on my head. Living with her is a window into my future.

She weighs seventy-seven pounds, not an ounce of fat, except for a boggy abdomen—the skin stretched from the three big babies her tiny frame bore—over which she can't bear to wear anything tight enough to stay up. Her long bony fingers, slightly crooked from mild arthritis, can overlap around her upper arm; two hands can easily wrap her thigh. She's always cold when it's so hot in the house I can barely function, dementia causing the brain to forget to tell the large muscles to be warm.

She is losing ground. But her heart keeps beating steadily behind her sagging flattened breasts; her lungs are still doing their job; her legs keep moving her unassisted inside the house, and anywhere else when there is a helping arm to steady and guide her; her mind remembers enough of what it needs to. She walks four laps four times a week around the tiny Lewis County mall, given over to social services offices except for Sears and a gun shop. She does deep knee bends holding onto the oven door handle. In the warm months, she walks on the deck and does arm lifts in the fresh air—if it's not so sunny that it hurts her eyes. Her body is wearing out, but it's not finished with its journey yet. And she isn't going to let it go as long as she has breath.

I marvel at her lack of inhibition in showing this body to me as I apply lotion after her shower. It is what she has to offer, and she does so without shame or modesty. It's the same body that ran home from grade school, stopping to pick a bouquet of the neighbor's flowers for her mother, that hiked the trails in the Smoky Mountains, that she joined with my father's as they conceived me, that rocked me to sleep, that held my babies and her first great-grandchild. She is not suffering from severe dementia; she would not throw off her clothes and walk out the front door. In fact, she rarely leaves her bedroom in her nightgown and bathrobe. Yet she offers her nakedness to my touch without a word or a grimace.

She is completely dependent on others to get her away from the house, to shop for the groceries she wants from her explicit lists, to remind her of things she refuses to admit she has forgotten. Books are no longer accessible to her except on tape from the Library for the Blind, played on a special player that can be slowed down and easily backed up so she can listen to a phrase or sentence over and over until she understands the words or gives up. Listening is exhausting, and she does so in small amounts. When she turns the player back on, she believes she has forgotten much of what has gone before, but she often has something to share with me over dinner.

She reads the newspaper with a magnifying glass a sentence or a paragraph at a time, with breaks. She listens to the TV news, but can't make out most of the words. She doesn't know what is on her dinner plate until she puts the food in her mouth or I tell her, and I've begun telling her what's there by position on a clock face. She says she can't see to write letters, though she continues to do so in perfectly chosen words—her perfect Palmer Method handwriting only just now becoming scraggly—expressing sympathy to friends and wives of my father's coworkers who have lost their spouse.

Although the team is large—family, caregivers, medical professionals, a few remaining elderly friends until one-by-one they die— each old person fights their own fight, alone against their body, on the last leg of the journey. I vow to double down in my efforts to respect the courage with which she walks this unchosen path and to be her advocate rather than her antagonist. I don't know why it's so hard.

20

January

Miracle, Not a Miracle

Michelle, her back issues resolved, came to the house today to ask Mama if she would like to hire her through Catholic Community Services, for regular times rather than as-needed and as-available. I overhear Mama tell her she needs to discuss it with me. It feels like a breakthrough.

"What do you think?" I ask when Mama tells me of the offer after Michelle leaves. I know her issue before she says it: paying for agency overhead, not understanding it includes worker benefits. I'm surprised she's considering it. "It will have to be regular times and hours," I remind her, not wanting her to say later she didn't know that, knowing she will say it anyway. "I think we should take her up on it, but the decision is yours. You like Michelle, and she knows how you like things done," I add, to plant a positive seed.

Mama ponders, then agrees to it. We decide on two-and-a-half hours a day, five days a week. In a moment of brain freeze, I tell myself I won't have to defend Michelle when Mama complains about her, since I didn't choose her.

The first day on the new schedule, Mama has forgotten Michelle is coming, and says she didn't realize she was coming five days a week.

After she leaves, I ask Mama how the morning was. "It was okay, I guess," she says. "I felt like I wasted the morning."

"What would you have done if Michelle hadn't been here?" I ask.

"I guess I would have tried to do what she did, but I wouldn't have gotten as much of it done." I try to discern the story behind the words, David's suggestion sinking in. Perhaps she feels more "worthless" (her word) when tasks get done without her. As long as it's not done, it's there waiting for her, and maybe tomorrow she will be able to do it herself. But aging is a pathway to the center of the labyrinth, with no return trip. My chest tightens. I don't want to be old.

❦

I return home late in the afternoon from Olympia to find Mama exhausted from having both Michelle and Stan here this morning. "They left at twelve thirty, and I didn't have lunch until two," she tells me.

"Didn't Michelle help you get your lunch before she left?" I ask, not bothering to offer again to help schedule Stan.

"I can get my own lunch, Gretchen," she snaps. She would rather be disappointed than give up control and independence.

❦

She begins to complain to me daily about Michelle's performance. I say nothing, even when she starts wanting to fire her and look for someone else.

Some days I feel myself turning and spiraling back toward the center of the labyrinth, falling into the patterns of this stranger with whom I am living, fearing I will become grouchy and pessimistic too. I go to the writing corner in the back of my father's workshop and sit in my favorite red leather armchair. I am infused with his presence as

I sit drinking in his optimism, his humor, his zest for life, wishing he were the one I was here with. *I will not become my mother*, I promise myself. *I will find the labyrinth's exit.*

I randomly find myself realizing I have nearly forgotten I used to have another life. A life in which I had a responsible job, where people counted on and appreciated me. I forget I had friends who loved me and a home of my own in which to bring them together, preparing a meal of my choosing that they raved about.

Just as random are days I accept that I again occupy the room where I slept and diagramed sentences and studied the periodic table as a teenager. I've had some good moments lately, when I feel kind and patient toward Mama. These are the times I sense I will get beyond the hard stuff and know I was a good daughter who enhanced the quality of the end of my mother's life.

But the good moments are sprinkled sparsely among the days and moments I think I can't do this anymore and I made a terrible mistake moving back here. I want to go home, except I am home. I don't want to repeat myself, trying alternate words to make Mama understand what I am saying. I don't want to tell her what's on her dinner plate that she can't see and watch her chase a bit of chicken around with her fork and then bring it empty to her mouth, making my heart break for her. I don't want to stop after every other sentence when I read to her to explain what she can't follow or to repeat a nonessential word. I want her to rejoice in what she can do instead of verbalizing the constant depression about what she can't that pulls me into the depths with her. I want to go to sleep without hearing her breathing over the buzzing baby monitor by my bed.

Tonight I want to sit on the sofa with my pizza and wine to watch the Golden Globes and not feel guilty that Mama is behind me eating alone at the table. And I want her not to choose the moment Jodie

Foster is speaking to join me in the living room to tell me she didn't call Michelle about new scheduling options this afternoon while I was away because she couldn't remember why she was supposed to call. I especially want her not to distract me while Jodie is poignantly talking about her mother who has dementia, hoping her mother is still there somewhere behind her blue eyes and will magically know in her soul that she is loved if Jodie tells her three times in a row.

"I love you," I tell Mama. "I'm glad I'm here with you."

"I love you too," she says. Tears well in her eyes and mine.

21

February

Health Care Battleground

Mama's story of how the "overdose" of medication in the hospital ruined her vision will surely join the family lore. The elderly, says Mary Pipher in her book *Another Country: Navigating the Emotional Terrain of our Elders*, don't suddenly develop bad personalities; they are overwhelmed by events. "It's post-traumatic stress," Pipher says. I listen to Mama telling yet another friend about it on the phone today, with new embellishments and changing the date from five months ago to mere weeks. Four doctors have told her the medication had no long-term effect, but she needs an explanation for ongoing deterioration, and this is what's available.

I am increasingly frustrated with the health care system. I take Mama to all kinds of specialists. She tells her bowel issues to her heart doctor, discusses her vision with the dermatologist, bemoans her lack of energy to her audiologist. Some of them listen patiently to her litany, others do not. She is desperate for someone who will care about her whole story.

May Sarton, who chronicled her advancing age in published journals, said hope dies last. Is this the clue to my mother's constant search for a cure for old age? She doesn't want drugs or surgery or physical therapy. She wants not to be old, and she tenaciously holds out hope that someone will wave a magic wand and save her. Talk is the only weapon she has in the battle, and she wants someone to listen and care—preferably someone with letters after their name—not just about her heart or her bones or her eyes or her stomach, but *her*.

Her cardiologists and primary care physician play hopscotch with her heart medication, increasing the dosage without consulting each other, decreasing it when Mama says it makes her tired, and then adding a second drug. Her long-time cardiologist, who is an ass, tells me if she is worried about her blood pressure he guesses I am going to have to get a monitor and "do some work." He has no clue what I do. I make her next appointment with his partner, who tells her if she doesn't have heart disease at her age, she isn't going to. "You have won the race!" he says. She doesn't believe him for a heart attack minute.

Eventually they will agree on the termination of both meds, along with the daily baby aspirin she self-prescribed when my father began taking it for his heart disease on doctor's orders—what's good for the gander. Mama will ignore them all and make her own decisions, self-medicating long after the prescriptions are eliminated, using up the bottles; changing the dosages herself to a level so low it wouldn't help if she did need them. Finally, she will abruptly announce she isn't taking them anymore, like it was her idea, saying "I think that's what's upsetting my stomach."

∾

We don't get a blood-pressure monitor. Lisa, Mama's new primary care provider, tells me sotto voce that Mama would drive me insane wanting to check it several times a day. Lisa and I are on the same page.

Rebecca and I talked Mama into trying Lisa, a physician assistant who introduced herself by her first name. Neither of us liked the doctor she had been going to for years. Mama couldn't understand his accent, and he didn't show any interest in her concerns. He talked to us rather than to her, which irritated all of us. We don't need to stick with what isn't working, now that there are two of us to break through Mama's inertia and the challenge of finding a provider taking new Medicare patients.

Mama likes Lisa: she is "thorough." She seems to know Mama wants to decide what she worries about—which is everything—and doesn't tell her not to. She takes time and answers all Mama's questions. She also doesn't say, "You're doing great for your age." Though she is, it's not what Mama wants to hear. I don't know what she does want to hear.

There are many caregivers out there in the strange unmapped land of this growing age group, and we have begun to find each other. Learning about being old-old in America—defined by gerontologists as over eighty-five—has become my passion. I add to my collection of books on aging research and inhale memoirs and blogs written by ordinary people caring for a parent. I turn my own bitchy private blog into a new public one that explores the landscape and hear from grateful readers, happy to know they are not alone and from whom I learn in turn.

"Old" comes at different ages. My mother was climbing a ladder to clean the flat roof of her home at eighty-five, while other people are using a cane at seventy. One day, I read, physicians will have standard tables to chart developmental progress of the elderly, perhaps based on things like hand-grip strength and lower body strength, just as they do with height and weight for children. Maybe then we will care for our eldest as well as we do our youngest.

∽

We have fallen back into stomach issues the past few days. I fear the onset of another crisis, my own PTSD kicking in. She is sure it was the half-serving of meatloaf she had two days ago that she had enthusiastically agreed to but now casts aspersions on because she "isn't used to a lot of beef." Or maybe it was the scallops Rebecca prepared at her request the day before that.

"I got sick on scallops several years ago," she says.

"When was that?" I ask, just before I bite my tongue.

"I visited George when he was in officer training in New York. I got scallops out of the Automat and spent the weekend sick in my hotel room."

"Ah. So around 1942?"

"My belly just doesn't feel normal," she says. She gives a Mona Lisa smile when I ask what normal would feel like, and admits it hasn't been normal for years. There's no point in suggesting that maybe this is her new normal; it's the surest way to motivate her to make yet another appointment with a specialist as she digs in her heels against my advice.

"I'm sorry," I say.

In my six months here, I have become desensitized to bowel discussions: whether or not they are moving, where she is when they do, and the quality and quantity of the output. She has been obsessed for decades, first keeping a journal in small spiral notebooks I find in a desk drawer, and more recently on scraps of paper I find all over the house. Now she gives me the daily report verbally.

These are the details that consume her attention nearly every moment. She talks about what she knows. Pipher says, "Illness is the battleground of old age. It is where we all make our last stand. That which cannot be talked about, cannot be put to rest." Would that talking about it would put it to rest. Then crisis comes in another form.

Without warning, powdered Metamucil disappears from the grocery and drugstore shelves. I'm skeptical that it works, but Mama thinks it does, and sometimes that's all that matters. I look in every store in Centralia and Olympia, and online. It's been recalled, the Target pharmacist finally tells me; she doesn't know when it will be back. We try wafers and chewable tablets, but they aren't what she's used to and therefore they don't work.

Mama is in a panic, and I make an appointment with Lisa, who recommends Miralax as a better alternative to Metamucil. Mama agrees to try it. It's a start. We'll see what Lisa is made of when Mama says it doesn't work.

We see Lisa again a week later for the results of her blood labs. Mama hopes they will tell her why her stomach is upset and her bowels sluggish all the time, and why she has no energy. She wonders if she is diabetic and needs to decrease sugar intake.

"I've stopped taking the Miralax," she tells me on the way to the office. "It upsets my stomach."

"Ah," I say, without argument. Lisa can deal with it. When she tells Lisa, Lisa says it is not causing stomach issues and it's the best thing to keep her bowels regulated, but she has to take it every day. I raise my eyebrows and say nothing. Neither does Mama.

"I never thought I would live this long," she tells Lisa. "I've had a good life, I don't need any more. But if I have to be here, I want to be healthy." It's a caveat I've heard many times. And so she eats the healthiest diet her digestive system will allow; she watches her cholesterol though her doctors tell her she won't live long enough for it to matter; she exercises; she avoids people who are sick and places where germs might lurk; she takes no risks lest she fall. And by clinging to control of all things she remains firmly tethered to this world through sheer will—if not enjoying her living.

She is far from home in an unfamiliar ocean on a sinking ship. What she is looking for is someone to get in the life raft with her. Perhaps when she tells people on the phone that the hospital robbed her of her vision, she is looking for someone who will at least pretend to share her outrage, which tells her that they care, that they will get in the raft. I wish I could just be grateful there is someone willing to listen to her, but I want to apologize to them for having to endure the stories and to tell them they aren't necessarily true. I want her not to sound crazy. I want her to let me steer the damn raft for her, but I'm not going to get in it without a paddle.

༄

We continue to make the rounds of primary care physician, cardiologist, ENT, audiologist, dermatologist, orthopedist, optometrist, glaucoma specialist, macular degeneration specialist, dentist, and podiatrist. And then we begin again. They all tell her the same thing: all is as well as it can be. Because there is no one who knows the whole story, she continues to tell each of them about issues outside of their specialty. No wonder managing their own healthcare is the full-time occupation of the elderly. No wonder adult children are exhausted caring for parents who can't care for themselves, especially when they believe they can.

When I'm an old-old—and this work is edging me there at lightning speed—I hope there are holistic clinics with health providers not pushing their own specialty as the only solution. I dream of referrals within the practice for yoga, physical therapy, chiropractic, mental health counseling, acupuncture, and naturopathy, as well as pharmaceutical and surgery options.

Changing the health care system is beyond my specialty, so I am my mother's health care manager. By the time this is done, I should have a degree. I'll settle for a tiara.

22

March

Escape

Without the framework of a job, the days slip by as rapidly as any day ever did, but it's hard to point to accomplishments. I didn't write anything other than a weekly blog post. I didn't change the gloom that settles over Mama. I didn't call a friend.

I read that when a person is under significant stress for a long period of time, the body floods with chemicals, becomes overwhelmed, and systems begin to shut down. It isn't only happening to Mama. I'm tired, anxious, short-tempered. I'm not burned out yet, but I'm slipping down the spiral behind her. I can't stop her slide, but I can take care of myself. Rebecca agrees to be on dinner and overnight duty, and I begin March with a leave of absence.

I spend a night with Emma and Wynne in Seattle, then drive to Bellingham for lunch with two writing friends. I stay in a bed and breakfast: wine, pizza, gas fire, book, a clawfoot bathtub, and blessed quiet. I forget to ask for the Wi-Fi password, which irritates me at first, but then I settle in and enjoy an evening off the grid. The next morning I drive over the border into British Columbia on a secondary road, for no other reason than I have a valid passport and a need to leave the claustrophobia of this life I have been inhabiting. I wish a passport were all I needed, but it's a start.

I drive along a narrow road on the US side, next to a water-filled ditch with an identical road on the Canadian side. I squint my eyes and imagine a different me on that side—living a different life. Which side is foreign? I'm not sure.

The Canadian border guard is not excited to let me in and wants to know why I'm not crossing at the interstate. Because I wasn't near the interstate. Because I prefer the road less traveled. I feel trapped and rejected as he finally waves me across, clearly believing he's letting an idiot into his country. I might as well be home doing things wrong in the kitchen.

~

I'm energized when I return home. The border guard wanted to know why I was entering his country, I'm determined to create a reason for being in my own. One that has to do with me, not with my mother. I register for a writers' meet-up group in Olympia. I submit a guest commentary to the local paper about being back in my hometown, and they publish it. I register for a drawing class at the local community college.

Emma tells me about a ten-hour-a-week job as communications manager for a small nonprofit in Seattle she saw online. Hoping it can be done remotely, I write a cover letter and send my resume. I'm called for an interview and offered the position. I say yes, after learning nearly all the work will be done from home. When I tell Mama I accepted it, she says, "Since you are doing so much for me, maybe you would rather do more instead of driving to Seattle so much. Michelle could cut back her hours and I could pay you instead."

I am glad to hear she recognizes I do a lot, but the thought of being her employee is a nightmare on steroids. "No, thank you," I say, managing to keep from guffawing. The job won't get me my independence back, but it will get me into the world again.

⌒∾

Last week we drew faces in my drawing class. I took a photograph of my mother as a young woman, the one my father took to Europe during the War. His "pin-up" girl he told his hut mates, so proud she had agreed to marry him. After my first attempt to draw it, the teacher says the eyes are really good. She says it's hard to draw people we know, we care too much that it be perfect. She helps me see where I went wrong. I begin again.

As I work, I see my mother when her whole life stretched before her. I glimpse in her eyes the woman who thought she would not find a forever love. When she hiked in a skirt with her girlfriends in the Smoky Mountains. When she worked behind the counter at the five and dime, hoping her monthly bleeding would not soak through the rags before she could get to the ladies' room during her prescribed brief break, and wearing her coat over her dress in case. I see in the set of her jaw the year she was in college and was told by her male professor that girls couldn't be missionaries—to China or anywhere else—and, giving up that dream, studied her bookkeeping lessons and Gregg shorthand by kerosene lantern light in her mother's boarding house. I see the young, ambitious woman, disappointed once more when she learned Tennessee didn't license female CPAs.

I see the hope in her eyes when she worked as the secretary to the boss at Tennessee Valley Authority and met my father when he came upstairs from his office to stand in the doorway of hers, and finally asked her out. I see the future in her not-quite smile before her lips met his for the first time. I see her courage when she moved around the country alone during the war years. I see the grit in her willing-ness to leave her beloved Tennessee mountains forever, moving to Washington to begin their life together.

I show her my drawing without telling her who my model had been. She doesn't recognize herself, and though the second one is better, neither do I. I continue to work on it deep into the inky night, Smudge sleeping on the sofa arm behind my head, and the rhythm of my mother's breathing coming through the baby monitor in the next room. I become obsessed with trying to catch the way the photog-rapher's light made her strawberry-blond hair translucent, hair her mother tied up in rags overnight to put a wave in it. I want to capture the enigmatic turn of her lips and the glint in her eye.

When I show it to Mama again she says the eyes are good.

23

April

Change of Plan

It's been a year since I accepted an offer on the sale of my house and began to pack in earnest.

I have done nothing in the nine months of my intended gap year toward working my way out of this situation. I suppose I settled in when Mama's well-being improved—whether or not she thought it had—with someone looking after her, or someone for her to look after.

Jo Ann comes out to be with Mama while I fly to North Carolina for a week of visits with family and friends. I don't drive by my house in Raleigh, afraid it will make me too sad. In Asheville, Ethan is ten months old; I missed his entire infancy. None of us can afford cross-country travel as my parents could when my children were young, flying us to Washington and themselves to us. It is a bittersweet trip, and I don't want to leave.

~

The day after my return, my sisters and I meet with an elder law attorney. I am concerned that Mama will live beyond the considerable savings she and my father planned well for. If she should have to apply for Medicaid—a government "hand out" she would throw herself in front of a train to avoid—we could lose the house after she dies. We learn we can avoid "repaying" a Medicaid debt with owned property if I live in the house with her for two years. Then it can be deeded to me, and I can deed one-third to each of my sisters, all tax-free. The thought of another year, with the first one not yet over, makes me queasy, but the bottom line is we aren't ready to move her, and I'm not prepared to move on. We decide to go for it; nothing will be lost if it works out differently.

"She won't agree to it," Rebecca says, as we call a family meeting before Jo Ann returns to Virginia. "She'll say she and Daddy planned that we were to sell the house and divide the money, not keep it."

"It was a long time ago," I say. "They didn't foresee the reality we are in now. We can't clean it out and sell it right now. And it will be ours when she dies anyway. This just ensures we will inherit it, not the government."

"That's true," Rebecca agrees.

"She is going to balk, though," I concur.

We decide to keep the Medicaid angle quiet—even though it's the biggest consideration—and focus on the fact that it will keep the property out of probate when she dies. She remembers that nightmare when our father died and wants to prevent us from dealing with it.

We sit around the table and Jo Ann, as eldest and the executor, explains what we have learned. She says we believe we should do it and asks Mama what she thinks.

"It would belong to all of us," I reiterate, "and it would still be yours to live in as long as it's feasible. Nothing would change."

"What do you think, Rebecca?" Mama asks.

"I think we should do it," she says, though I get the feeling her heart isn't in it.

"Who would pay the taxes and upkeep?" she asks.

"Your estate would continue to pay everything," Jo Ann says. "It's still your house."

We sit quietly then, holding our collective breath while she ponders.

"Okay," she says. "I'm glad you are staying, Gretchen. And I'm glad you all love this place." I'm not sure her heart is in it either.

We are stunned it was so easy. I'm stunned at what I just agreed to. Fourteen months feels more solid and thereby longer than the unspecified duration when she told David she wanted to stay at home.

∽

I toss and turn night after night, unable to fall asleep, or waking at two in the morning, my mind racing. Is this what losing your mind feels like?

Six years ago, Rebecca and I traveled to Tanzania to visit Emma in the Peace Corps. At the end of our visit, we boarded a small ferry on the Indian Ocean under blue skies to travel from Zanzibar to Dar es Salaam where we would board our plane to head home. The sky turned black as soon as we left port, and a fierce storm accompanied our crossing, with most of the passengers vomiting into bags the entire voyage. We traveled parallel to the coast, which sometimes could be seen and mostly could not, as the boat pitched and rocked. I have never been so scared, or felt so trapped. Until now.

Sometimes I dare to visualize a future when Mama isn't here, or I'm not, but I can't imagine abandoning her, sending her to a facility or hiring full-time care. She isn't adapting well to her very part-time caregiver; how can I relegate her to nearly exclusive care by someone else?

This is my life for now, I remind myself during the wakeful nights.

I need to keep swimming, parallel to the shore until I get to calmer waters. One day I will be able to turn toward land and get back on terra firma. *I will not drown. I will not drown.*

Four hundred fifty-seven days to go. At least.

24

April

Talking About the Inevitable

I submit beneficiary forms for Mama's bank and investments accounts. The transfer of deed is executed and will be filed next July. If she lives until then, there will be nothing to go through probate when she dies. We update her simple will and make sure all legal documents are in order. Copies of powers of attorney are in an envelope to take to the hospital whenever she goes. Getting legal and financial matters in order is my biggest accomplishment to date.

We move on to health matters, completing Washington's advance directive and the Physician Orders for Life Sustaining Treatment (POLST) that goes on her refrigerator or bedroom door for EMTs, with a copy in the hospital envelope. It is surprisingly easy to discuss her end-of-life wishes. She is nearly ninety-seven; she won't die prematurely. It feels like she has been waiting for the conversation that I had been reluctant to bring up, fearing I was rushing her. It's not uncommon for children to think it will be too hard for the parent and parents to think it will be too hard for the children, and so it too often stays unspoken and unprepared for.

She does not want life-sustaining measures taken. Comfort only. Except that, well, her mother. At ninety-nine, she needed a blood transfusion—not for the first time—in order to stay alive. My parents were visiting family on the other side of the country when the doctor called. My mother told him no heroic efforts—enough was enough, I suppose—then got on a plane for home. She was not in time.

"My mother died alone. It still haunts me," she tells me across the dining room table, her voice catching on a sob of rare emotion as my pen hovers over the form.

"It may have been what she wanted," I say gently. "People do that. They wait until they are alone and then they let go. She was a loner in life and in death." Mama is quiet, lost in her grief and regret that she let her mother down, unable to hear my words or trust my compassion.

"And so did George," she adds softly. She had just left the hospital that June day in 1995, and returned home, when they called her to come back. Nicholas had been here visiting, and was helping his papa replace the fence around the meadow when my father began having chest pains. Nicholas, with a brand-new driver's license, took him to the hospital, my mother out shopping and blissfully unaware. Three days later, on the longest day of the year, it was Nicholas who returned his nana there when the nurse called. My father had a massive heart attack and died before they arrived.

I'm silent then too, tears leaking from my eyes, remembering his death, the event a triad with Father's Day and my birthday. He was angry with me over my divorce, and we hadn't spoken since the last time I had seen him, at Thanksgiving, both of us too proud to break the silence. When he finally called, on my birthday, I wasn't home. He was rude to my partner on the phone, and I didn't call him back. The next evening, moments after returning from a walk on which I observed for the first time—and to date, the last—the synchronous blue light dance of thousands of mating fireflies, my mother called to tell me he was "gone." He had died as I stood in awe watching the fireflies. At a family gathering months later, as I wept in my grief that I had missed that call, that we were estranged when he died, Jo Ann tells me she always thought the firefly dance had been a spirit moment of reconciliation. Over the years, I've had several dreams that healed the breach. I hear my mother's own regrets, now, of what didn't happen at the end of his life or her mother's.

"Are you afraid to be alone when you die?" I ask.

"No," she says, "I just don't want my children to feel bad for decades like I have. I don't want to make that choice for you."

I don't hang onto regrets like she does, so it's unlikely that I will be guilt-ridden for decades, but after I check "no life-sustaining measures" on the POLST, I write in that her daughters are free to override the directive and she initials it. I expect that is understood by medical and legal professionals, but specifying it dispels Mama's qualms.

Stellajoe E. Staebler, she writes in her newly wavery handwriting next to my finger, showing her the signature line. I feel like she just signed her own death warrant. I wonder if she feels it.

25

May

Another Scare

When I come upstairs this morning, Mama is standing at the counter cutting spinach for her scrambled eggs.

"Good morning," I say.

The words are barely out of my mouth when the knife clatters to the floor as she grabs her head and leans over the counter, moaning low and steady.

My heart stops beating. "What's happening?" I cry.

The moans increase in pitch and volume as I slip my arms under her armpits to keep her from collapsing.

"Don't hold me so tight!" she screams.

"Let me help you get to the chair," I say calmly, though my heart is pounding now.

"Let go!" she shouts.

Supporting her as gently as I can, I snag the ladder-back chair at the built-in desk with my foot and pull it over. She sits down, still holding her head and groaning. When her head lightly grazes my arm behind it, she screams, "Don't squeeze my head!"

And then it's over, three minutes. She insists she is fine and returns to her breakfast prep. I'm shaking.

I call Rebecca and tell her what happened. "It scared the crap out of me," I say. "Do you have time to go have coffee when Michelle gets here?"

"I'll make time," she says.

An hour later, over lattes at Santa Lucia, I tell her my fears. "It's another wake-up call, like the strained back a few months ago. We're not ready for her future. How many warnings does she have to give us?"

Rebecca nods. "You know, I think about how Mama was Daddy's caregiver through his heart events and the angioplasty, as much as he would allow her to 'give care,' and that was enough. If they thought about his needing more care in the future, I never heard about it. And then he was building the fence one day, and that evening he was in the hospital, and three days later he was dead."

"Right," I say, "and we're just going along like that's what will happen with Mama, and we know damn well it's not how it's going to go down with her. She could have a stroke or a fall, and we aren't prepared for that level of caregiving. We've got to have a plan and her name on waiting lists for skilled nursing care."

Rebecca agrees, but I know she is busy. Jo Ann is far away. I suffer from "cross that bridge when we get to it" syndrome, when it will be too late for a bridge. We wonder if the event was a TIA—a transient ischemic attack, sometimes called a mini-stroke—but we don't have her checked out. Maybe we should have, but there will be no intervention, and we don't need a roadmap for a journey we aren't going to take. I fear she will continue this gradual decline accompanied by small events until something far more catastrophic than death happens and, in our unpreparedness, we are knocked to our knees.

26

May

Old Story

A few days after the kitchen scare, Mama tells me she woke up early and should have gotten up; then her head wouldn't be full of things she didn't need to be thinking about.

"Like what?" I ask, wondering if she worries about having a stroke, if the recent incident felt like a harbinger, if she even remembers it.

"Like the hospital robbing me of my vision," she says. "I need to write a letter, then maybe I can let it go."

"Let's do it then," I say, beyond ready to put the lorazepam incident to rest.

Two days later, she asks me to type what she wrote. It's almost entirely fiction. She accepts my offer to rewrite it for her, but I don't have a clue where to begin. Events from several hospital visits over the years are woven with the most recent visit in late September. She has added a phantom experience "in December or January" that she claims is the one that "robbed" her. She once told me her boss at a long ago job accused her of trying to make him look bad when she—determined to make him look better than he was—corrected the letters he dictated to her. It saddens me to hold in my hand the evidence that my brilliant mother, writer of many intelligent letters to the editor of the local newspaper and other publications, is no longer in charge of her brain.

"Do you want me to include your perceptions of what happened even though they aren't true?" I ask her.

"Yes," she says without hesitation, not because she wants me to lie, but because she believes my version of the event is seriously flawed.

I try to make the letter as accurate as possible so she doesn't sound like a crazy person, while slanting the truth to accommodate her story. I include words like "I believe" to her statement that she was given an overdose of lorazepam, and "my glaucoma specialist told me the medication 'could' have caused blindness," rather than "confirmed" that it did. What he really said was "it could have temporarily contributed to blurry vision," but I know the full truth won't fly with her. I give her the result, after running drafts by Rebecca for her knowledge of past events, and hold my breath.

She says it is beautifully done. I exhale.

∾

When I come upstairs for breakfast the next morning, she greets me with, "You have to change the letter. There are some things in it I don't remember happening because I was out of it. For instance you said you put your phone numbers on the board in the room. I'm afraid if the letter doesn't say, 'I was told that . . .' it will make the complaint unbelievable, because how could I know that if I wasn't conscious, as I claim?" It's almost a rational thought process, except we put our numbers on the board before she had the medication.

She also insists I put back in that she was given three little pink pills (lorazepam) and a white one (metoprolol). I don't point out those were the things that allegedly happened when she was "out of it," nor do I tell her again that it couldn't have happened because she was on a nothing-by-mouth order, and they wouldn't have administered her heart medication at midnight in any case. All she remembers are the things she has imagined. I do as she asks, sad and embarrassed for her, and for myself as an accessory.

∽

A few weeks after the letter is mailed, the hospital calls. Mama can't understand what the woman is saying and calls me to the landline. The nursing supervisor is apologetic about the incident. Trying not to discredit Mama and her very real trauma following the event, I tell her I realize some of what she said in the letter came out of hallucinations—that were, perhaps, caused by the lorazepam. I emphasize the two things I believe to be where they erred: they didn't call her daughters when there was a change in her condition as we expressly requested, and it didn't seem like they took her age and weight into account in the dosage. I also question if her record reflected that she had shown no agitation at all the day before, or if the staff even looked at her record.

I hang up the phone and sit down next to Mama, waiting in the chair at the dining room table near the phone.

"She's very sorry for your experience. She promises she will give a report to the staff and that they will look at their policies and procedures when dealing with elderly patients and their families."

"Good," Mama says.

"You've been an advocate for better care. Your activist days are not over, are they? Maybe it will make a difference."

"I just hope because of my experience no one else will have to go through what I did," she says.

With the resolution, she has become a woman without a story. Or so I think.

⌒

Five days after the phone call, we drive to Seattle to see the glaucoma specialist. Dr. M is Mama's third doctor in this office. Though very young, she is one of the most compassionate, patient, understanding doctors I have seen, speaking directly to Mama and saying helpful things clearly. After telling the technician the lorazepam story, she says nothing to Dr. M.

"The steady decline in your vision is consistent with the combination of glaucoma and macular degeneration you have," Dr. M says.

"Is it a typical decline or could a trauma hasten it?" I ask, being sure Mama can hear me.

"You mean the medication she received in the hospital?" Dr. M asks. The technician must have put it in her record, and Dr. M must actually have read it.

"Yes," I say.

Leaning closer and looking straight at Mama, she says what the previous specialist told her, but less dismissively, "The drug did not make your vision worse. Hospitals are always stressful places and the stress could have affected your vision temporarily. Even the medication could have affected it while it was in your system. But when the drug left your system, your vision would have recovered completely to what it had been." She pauses to let that sink in. "The memory of a sudden loss at that moment is likely what you are recalling, but it was declining steadily before that and has continued to decline steadily. It did not change your vision."

Mama is silent. I doubt she will absorb that, or trust it, because Dr. M isn't her familiar doctor, but the clarity helps me understand.

⌒

After lunch, we go on to the low vision clinic.

"How are you today, Stellajoe?" the doctor asks. I hold my breath.

"Well," Mama says with a pregnant pause. "Not too good. I had to spend some time in the hospital and they gave me an overdose of lorazepam and now I can't see."

The top of my skull lifts right off my head.

The reason we are back here is to work again with the idea of reading glasses. Last time Mama was so discouraged she said the test lens didn't help because it didn't make it "easy" to read—at least that's my theory. I suggested on the drive up that she keep her mind open and positive, look for "better" and let go of "perfect."

With the reading lens, she reads four lines smaller than with her usual glasses. I'm so excited for her.

"Would you like to try reading glasses?" the doctor asks.

"I don't know," Mama says.

♄

On the way home I ask her if she would like to get the prescription I insisted on filled.

"I don't know if it's worth it," she says. "Maybe I just need to move somewhere I can get full-time care." Then she says, softly, "You need to get on with your life."

"This is my life right now," I say. She tears up a bit, and no more is said.

27

May

Dreaming of the Future

It was a single sentence. It may change my life. I'm reading *The Dirty Life: On Farming, Food, and Love*, a memoir by Kristin Kimball about a city girl who becomes a farmer and, with her new husband, starts a farm cooperative. "The central question in the kitchen," she writes, "would have to change from 'What do I want?' to 'What is available?'"

The sentence jumps off the page, and I bolt upright in my chair. I have been asking myself what I want next. I have explored towns I might want to live in, rejecting most of them and having reservations about others. I have pondered a return to piecing together jobs to support my living and worried in advance that I won't be able to afford to live anywhere I would want to be. I signed on to another year with Mama partly because I didn't know what else to do. Then comes this question, "What is available?"

What is available is this property my sisters and I grew up on. This home I am currently living in. This place my parents nurtured and my children love. I have wondered what my sisters and I could do with it—other than sell it for an unworthy price in this economically depressed county—but I haven't taken it very seriously because

131

the thought of staying in this town feels more like surrender than adventure, more like a fallback than a plan. And I haven't felt confident that I have the desire or the ability to invest the energy it would take to turn it into a business venture.

But maybe the right vision just hadn't come along. The vision that could persuade me to give up some of what I thought I wanted next: to live nearer to grandchildren and make a home where I can walk to places I need to be. When we choose one thing, we must say goodbye to something else. All at once I feel a long-absent surge of energy and excitement.

I walk up to the meadow in search of sun, which doesn't hit the house in the early hours. I sit in the barn doorway, looking out over the dew-covered meadow as the fog gives way. The sun warms my face as it rises over the neighbor's apple orchard and the towering noble firs my father planted as seedlings across the driveway.

I sip my coffee and let the thoughts float through my head as the mist floats over the meadow. *What is it that you most want? What drove you to move back here? What is the underlying desire?* I wanted to return to the Northwest and to know and be known by my family. Just those two things. All else is open.

As I sit, ideas begin to swirl. A retreat center, a Golden Girls home with friends, a tiny house in the meadow for me. I had been looking at this property as a tired part of my past. Now suddenly I see it as a gift to be unwrapped. I see possibility, not only to do a new thing in my life, but to breathe new life into this place on the hill. It's a link to the past with a hope for the future.

I gaze across the sparkling meadow. My father had a garden here once—mostly corn and squash. I begin to visualize my own garden in this sun-drenched meadow. I could grow vegetables for the family and maybe enough to share with the neighbors. I imagine an enclosure not only to keep out deer and rabbits, but creative; not only vegetables, but flowers. A place for retreatants to sit and meditate or write. A labyrinth appears in the corner of the meadow. I close my eyes. I am walking the path that weaves in toward my mother and back out toward my Self, in and out, in and out. Passing her and leaving her, as she steadily makes her way to the center.

Am I considering staying here indefinitely, turning the one year, and now two, into forever? And perhaps keeping Mama with me as long as she is able? I survived four years in Mississippi, the angst of coming out as a lesbian, the end of two important relationships, learning to live on my own again, buying my own house, and leaving that house. And now I'm contemplating the greatest challenge of all: staying in a relationship with my mother until death do us part.

28

May

Living in the Present

I decide not to tell anyone my idea yet, afraid of scaring it off. I may never tell Mama. She will be full of unsolicited reasons for its impossibility: the septic tank, respect for the neighbors, security, it's my sisters' house too. She will pick up her "we have to sell the house" mantra. It's not time to think about why it won't work. I know she believes she has my best interests at heart, that she doesn't want me saddled with the upkeep like she has been, that it's her last responsibility to her children to keep that from happening, overlooking her own admission that being here gave her purpose when she found herself alone.

I'm almost twenty years younger than my mother was when my father died. I still have adventure in me. I've been flying solo for nearly a decade. I know how it's done; I know how to look ahead for what might be coming. I am trusting myself that I will know when it's time to leave and that I will be able to do it. I may be delusional, but I have made difficult decisions in my life—seemingly impossible decisions—and they always come out right enough.

I take a previously scheduled two-day getaway. It's perfect timing. I hang out in Seattle at a friend's home on the edge of Puget Sound, sitting with my big idea, watching the sun set over the water and the ferries, barges, and eagles pass back and forth. I could do this. Excitement rises up in me, and I feel a surge of resolve to care better for my mother while I wait for my time to come.

⌒

The morning after my return I come upstairs, and Mama greets me with, "I need spinach, chard, or kale every day."

"Good morning," I say.

"And I can't eat fried food." I assume she is constipated. I can't fix that, she won't take her Miralax regularly. And I never fry food, but I know she means sautéed.

"And I guess I'll have to curtail my laundry because other people do too much," she says, moving on. "The septic system can't take it."

I've been gone, and it upset her apple cart.

"I do one load of laundry every other week," I say, diving into the morning's rabbit hole. "I don't know how I can do less. You might have to take up the issue with Rebecca who does more than I do, and she doesn't even live here," I add, throwing my sister under the bus. I don't engage in her paranoia about the septic system.

⌒

When I put dinner on the table this evening, Mama asks what the fish du jour is.

"Sole," I say.

"What kind of sole?"

"Dover, as instructed," though only because that's what they had. I was going to get whatever I found and bury the label in the wastebasket as usual.

"How did you cook it?" she asks.

"Baked. In a parchment bag with minced carrots, onions, and red peppers. Served with lemon dill sauce." Sounds like a restaurant menu.

"I don't think I can eat it," she says.

There has been no success in the bathroom in too long. We discuss bodily function over dinner, getting to the bottom of the morning complaints. She wonders if it is one of the medications she is taking.

"I should have gone to the drugstore and gotten a printout of side effects."

"You have a file folder full of them, plus it's online. Just ask me."

"But I haven't read them, have you?"

"Yes, and I have read them to you."

"What do they say?" she challenges.

"All medications list constipation or diarrhea as possible side effects." I try to think of a change of subject, but I'm not fast enough.

"What kind of spinach is this?" she asks. "I can only eat baby spinach."

"I used what you and Michelle bought. I know better than to buy adult spinach."

We finish eating in silence then, spent. She cleans her plate.

∾

I call Rebecca in tears when I go downstairs for the night. It took every tool in my kit to get through the dinner complaints. My two days away are distant memory. Rebecca says it's not my job to please Mama.

"That's not what she thinks," I say. "Why can't she say she's sorry that after I went to so much effort she doesn't feel like eating tonight, instead of making it my fault?"

"I don't know. It's her version of dementia. It doesn't matter what she thinks, anyway; you know you are loving her well. Ignore her words."

"Is that what you would do?" I ask skeptically.

"No," she admits. "And I'm not there on the front line. I'm worried about you."

Her concern is genuine, but I hear it as I'm a whiny bitch and becoming unpleasant to be around. It's how I see myself.

I feel I'm doing nothing of value other than cooking Mama's dinner—however unsatisfactorily. David, consultant and champion, reminds me I make her living possible. I am her eyes, showing her the world. I am the keeper of routines and organizational structure that keep her together and able to function. I give her the confidence to continue living "alone." I provide her the illusion she is still in control.

We are both going to have good days and bad days, I tell myself as I lie in bed waiting for sleep. Smudge curls up on my legs, not a great substitute for someone's arms around me tonight, but I'll take her comforting presence. Mama will continue to challenge me, and maybe one day I will learn how to deal with it. In any case, we will navigate this labyrinth together until her path dead-ends and mine opens to the future and whatever it holds.

I drift off to sleep, not dreaming of the future, but wondering what I will cook for dinner tomorrow.

29

June

New Life

I've been here through the four seasons and learned what each has to offer: foggy dawns, the bluest blue and the greyest grey skies, all-day rain and bone-chilling damp, spectacular flowers, crisp cool mornings and hot afternoons, rainbows, and spectacular sunrises over the valley.

Today is Mama's ninety-seventh birthday; my own birthday is in two weeks and Rebecca's a week after mine. I never thought this was where I would find myself at sixty-one. In the past two decades, though, I have accepted that life comes as it will.

Emma and Wynne come down for the weekend to celebrate our three birthdays. Emma, who landed a job as soon as she arrived in Seattle with a nonprofit providing services for youth experiencing homelessness, has moved up the organizational ladder. Wynne is in graduate school finishing a master's degree in education. Their lives are full, and I'm grateful when they steal a precious weekend for a visit.

We all sit around the table in Rebecca's apartment in the back of her shop eating the dinner she prepared, then blowing out candles, opening gifts, and eating chocolate cake.

"One more gift, for all of you," Emma says as we finish, pulling a small tissue-wrapped package out of her lap and handing it to me.

I tear off the tissue paper, and gasp.

It's a tiny T-shirt printed with the words, "Gigi moved for me." After a breath-held moment, I burst into tears. Emma and Wynne, teary too, get up and hug me.

"Emma is pregnant!" Rebecca explains to Mama.

"Oh! That's wonderful!" Mama exclaims, clutching her hands to her chest, her eyes filling too. If she wonders how that could happen with two women, she doesn't ask. "When?"

"In eight months," Emma says.

In February, there will be a baby. I'm barely breathing. Caring for my mother is only one of the reasons I came here. Some days it feels like my whole life, but it's not. And it's temporary. A grandchild is forever.

∼

The summer solstice, the day after my birthday, is the eighteenth anniversary of my father's death. The summer and winter solstices have long been my favorite days of the year, gateways into a new season. I watch the sunrise from my bed and wonder what my second summer here will bring. As I begin to look after some things on this property myself, I am more in awe of my mother. How in the world did she care for it all, in her eighties, alone?

I make pancakes for breakfast, with apples as my father made them—Saturday morning pancakes being his only ventures into the kitchen. As we sit down to eat, trying not to let the light- and view-blocking window shades depress me, I broach my curiosity.

"What was it like for you to take care of all of this without Daddy?"

"Well," Mama says hesitantly, "I waited until something needed to be attended to, and then I dealt with it. Usually I called someone."

I'm hoping to hear how she dealt with it emotionally. I press her: "Did you feel overwhelmed? Did you despair? Did you cry?"

"I just did what had to be done, one day at a time. I should have gotten out of here right away, but I didn't. And it gave me something to do."

I wonder if she would still be alive if she'd left this house, garden, and history on the hill. It gave her purpose, a big factor in longevity. She was seventy-nine years old when my father died, too young to need care, too old to start over, a woman ensconced in place. Always fiercely independent, she didn't talk to any of us about moving to a progressive care facility instead of staying in the house, and we didn't raise the subject. She never told us about problems, and I never asked how she was doing, if it was too much, how I could help. I was wrapped up in my own life three thousand miles away. If I have regrets, it's not that I'm not doing enough now, but that I didn't attend to her grief back then.

I see now, though, her continuing hold on independence—pretending she doesn't need help and not wanting to "bother" me—was as true then as it is now. She doesn't understand it would be easier to be asked for help than to guess at what she needs; my offers of assistance strip her of self-reliance. Is acceptance of what one can no longer do a kind of courage? And asking for help a kindness? We need a new paradigm.

∾

After breakfast, I walk up to the meadow and sit in the barn door with my journal. It's become my favorite summer thinking post. *My mother has given me a gift*, I write, *a crystal ball to my own elderhood, and the opportunity to shape my future and my relationship with my daughter differently. To be the revered elder, not the exasperating elder-ly.* I laugh out loud. I'm sure I will still be exasperating. I hope I will be able to acknowledge it.

Lifting the pen, I watch a deer come into the meadow from across the driveway. I saw her baby a few days ago and wonder where it is.

When I began to get serious about moving here, Emma—perhaps not jokingly—suggested I could provide childcare when they had children. "Uh no," I said then, "been there done that." Now I can't wait for the opportunity to build a relationship with this child, and to establish a new place in the family. I pick up my pen again.

What if we banished the dichotomy of dependent versus independent? What if we embraced the fact that we all need other people at all stages of life? What if we are all always dependent and always independent? Interdependent.

The fawn bounds across the driveway and takes its place next to its mother, who lifts her head briefly, then resumes grazing.

This "do it myself" insistence was not always so, I realize, watching the deer, my mind wandering from the page again. The generations used to care for one another. My family, though, has had a wanderlust since WWII, my parents leaving home and moving across the country, my sisters and I reversing the directional migration. And yet, here are Rebecca and I, back again. And here is my own daughter, about to become a mother on the other side of the continent from where she was raised. Four generations living, if not quite together, at least close enough to be in relationship. We are already doing a new thing.

year two

30

July

Respite

In celebration of the anniversary of my arrival, I've planned a camping trip. I savor my euphoria of anticipation as long as I can before I tell Mama I'm going to Mt. Adams while Jo Ann and Peter are here. When I finally break the news, she is full of the expected negativity: "There won't be any huckleberries yet." "Is anyone going with you?" "Don't you think it's dangerous to go camping alone?" "It will be dry and hot." I assure her I will be fine, knowing she is not reassured.

The day arrives, the car is packed, and I am raring to go, departing as soon as everyone is out of bed, leaving it all in Jo Ann's hands. My destination is Takhlakh Lake, a remote campground in the Gifford Pinchot National Forest. In miles, it's not so far away, but distance in the wilderness is measured not in miles, but in time it takes to traverse forest roads, including several miles of bone-rattling washboard gravel surface and pothole dodging. There is no cell phone service, no electricity, no potable water, and no flush toilets. I'm in heaven.

The lake is ringed by tall, straight Douglas fir, flocked with dripping pale yellow lacy lichen. Spring-green grasses grow at water's edge, and huckleberry bushes, still a month or more from fruiting, fill the forest. The mountain, the trees, wispy clouds, and in the evening the moon double their glory in lake reflection.

Mist hovers at the surface of the lake as dawn breaks the first morning. I sit in my chair above the water's edge, watching and listening. It is utterly still. The first rays of the sun still hidden behind the trees dazzle the snow on the side of the mountain peak. The *kaflop kaflop* of a young osprey's wings breaks the silence as it circles the lake above the mist in search of breakfast. It flies, disappointed, into a treetop after failing at instant success; the lake reclaiming silence, save for the plopping of fish jumping for joy.

My red REI insulated coffee mug empty, I return to my campsite to cook eggs and bacon.

∽

When I return to the lakeside with my breakfast, a large male osprey is on the scene, his broad beautiful wings silent as he circles at treetop level, searching. Unlike his young predecessor, he glides tirelessly, up and back and across the lake, soaring higher, swooping lower. Abruptly, with a quick twist of the body and a flash of white belly, he dives straight down. Milliseconds before impact he aborts and flaps back to a treetop height vantage point as the prey gets away. The pattern continues with several more dives. Only once does he splash into the water, apparently missing the lightning-quick fish.

For more than an hour I watch enthralled, not turning away until my eye catches the sideshow. Mama and baby wood duck paddle back and forth in front of me. Suddenly Mama dives under the water and is gone. Baby, oblivious to her disappearance, continues to paddle on. Mama resurfaces and, deep in her throat, calls to her wayward child.

The baby turns its head and possibly rolls its eyes; then, with no sense of urgency, heads back her way.

In the moment I am distracted by the ducks, the osprey flies over me from behind, a fish in his talons. I heard nothing: no splash, no squeal from the doomed fish, no *creee creee creee* from the hunter trumpeting his victory. I'm sorry I missed the snatch, and grateful to have borne witness to the patient hunt and the reward.

I want to be like the mature osprey, sticking with Mama, not giving up, knowing I will miss the mark many times until I finally get it right. And I guess I am. Maybe I'm too hard on myself.

My mind drifts to my childhood, when Mama was the mother duck, I the child. She let me stray back then. I had an idyllic childhood at the edge of one of the southern fingers of Puget Sound, where we lived the first eight years of my life. I would dash out the back door on summer mornings, letting the wooden screen door slam behind me, run across the lawn, past the lattice fence covered with my mother's trailing roses, and into the woods that bordered the mud flat at low tide. I played there all day, in my memory, savoring the independence she seemingly allowed me. She called me home for meals, a reminder of her care for me. She taught me to trust myself. She was not always afraid, or she hid it better. Who she is now is not her essence.

Each day, the early morning hours on the lake belong to the mountain, the birds and fish, the misty dawn and the rising sun, a solitary angler or two in silent boats, and me. Friday afternoon—the day of my departure—brings an onslaught of recreation seekers, weekend campers, and loud picnickers. I break camp and pack the car, leaving the lake to them.

I wish I could stay forever. I know I will be back. I bounce back over the gravel road, swerving around the potholes, occasionally falling into one. It isn't lost on me that my life with my mother is like this road.

It's been 365 days. The end is not in sight, and there will be many more potholes. I will fall into some of them and skirt the edge of others. I return home thinking, *Maybe I can do it. Be the osprey.*

31

September

I Can't

"How do you make syrup?" Mama asks one morning, after standing motionlessly at the stove for several moments as I make pancakes. I'm startled; it's a simple process she's done all her life. I throw out suggestions, and it comes back to her. It's one of the first clear indicators of something beyond simple memory loss.

While the admission of mental diminishment is rare, she reminds me several times a day that her vision is fading to nothingness. "Is there mold on that loaf of bread? I can't see." "I can't find my hearing aid remote; is it on the table? I can't see." "Did I get my signature on the line? I can't see." It's attached to every third sentence out of her mouth. What does she want? Sympathy? Acknowledgment? Does reminding me—and herself—that she can't see trick her into believing it's not her brain that's failing? As the world fades from her vision, maybe she feels like she is fading into a ghost, invisible to the world.

∽

When we sit down for dinner tonight, I look out the window for the first time since morning and gasp at the presence of the mountain. She has been veiled for several days behind the overcast skies and last weekend's heaviest September rainfall in history. She has a new coat of snow, and the setting sun has her in its golden spotlight.

I remember not to tell Mama to look; instead describing the spectacle to her. She turns her head to the east and quickly back to her plate and the business at hand. "I can't see it," she says.

The familiar words snatch the breath out of me. "Are you able to verbalize why you constantly need to remind yourself and everyone else that you can't see?" I'm both curious and frustrated.

"I guess because people believe I can see more than I can."

"I don't think that's the case," I say. "And what difference does it make if they do? I wonder if constantly reminding yourself of what you can't do might be increasing your depression and your belief that you are worthless."

Using too many words, as I do when I'm frustrated, I continue, "You've lived here for fifty-three years and taken hundreds of pictures of the mountain in all kinds of light. You know what it looks like. Maybe when I describe it, you could say, 'I can imagine it!' or 'It sounds beautiful,' or 'Thank you for sharing it with me.' Every time you say 'I can't see,' you're giving a piece of your world away. What if you focused on what you *can* do?" It's a pretty good speech.

"Would you rather I blame you?" she asks.

"What do you mean?" I ask, confused. She says nothing. Is she using her loss of vision to explain her depression to avoid blaming me for that? Blaming me for being here keeping her alive? Most likely she has no more idea what she meant than I have. "It isn't about me," I say, "it's about the message you send to yourself and how it makes you feel about your life." She is silent.

She has always had a low self-image, despite her courage. She survived a challenging childhood that would have broken many people, moved alone back and forth across the country during the war, participated in national peace efforts and advocated for gun control, spearheaded the movement to save the trees on this hill, and kept up her home largely alone for the past eighteen years. It's not only glaucoma and macular degeneration that limit her vision, but the tightly gripped "I can't" story she has told herself for so long—and been told by a male-dominated society, particularly in her generation—that she is blind to any other.

Sometimes I remove my glasses and close one eye and squint through the other, trying to imagine her experience. I wonder if I would even get out of bed in the morning.

Like Helen Keller's breakthrough under Annie Sullivan's tutelage, a few days later, Mama says, "Maybe I should concentrate on what I am able to do."

"Good idea!" I say, as if it were hers. I am determined to mold her into the cheerful, optimistic mother I want her to be.

∾

In the next days, she seems to be trying to remember her vow. Several times I sense "I can't see it" ready to come out, then not hit the airwaves. But I overhear her pausing when she is talking to others, as if considering whether to let the words slip out, and then is unable to resist the temptation.

At the dinner table one night, I test her. I tell her the sky to the east is still grey and foggy, as it has been all day, but the setting sun in the west has found its way through the clouds and is shining down the valley and lighting up the red barn on the other side. She turns to look and says, "All I see down there is light."

I remain calm, saying, "I know you can't see it with your eyes. Close them and try to see it in your mind."

"I have seen it many times, I can imagine it," she says.

"Yes!" I say.

"Thank you for describing it," she says. Maybe she means it, maybe she is mollifying me. It doesn't matter; it's a start.

32

November

Thursdays with Mama

Thursdays, when Michelle doesn't come, is the day I designated—before I knew better—to spend doing Mama's bidding. Today is too stormy for an outing and we have no doctor appointment, which means we are staying in again, doomed to another task that will challenge my patience. It's just one day, I tell myself. Maybe I can help it be a happy one.

Over breakfast of scrambled eggs with sautéed red peppers and chanterelle mushrooms, bacon, warmed fruit compote, and homemade blueberry ricotta coffee cake from the freezer, I take a deep breath and ask what she wants to do today. She is ready with an answer.

"Michelle was looking for fabric to re-cover my rice bag and couldn't get to the boxes on the shelves in the storeroom because of all the stuff on the floor in front of it. I just had her get the first one she came to, which wasn't what I wanted. I want to clean up the area in front of the shelves."

I sigh. I know it isn't going to be only the pathway she has her sights set on, and I wonder what subterfuge I can use to get stuff out of the house, not merely rearranged.

The room is a disaster. Besides the bloated cupboards where

I continue to shift things to make room for more, an army trunk under the table holds my grandmother's unfinished quilt tops and fabric scraps from clothes she made for me and my sisters, including an empire waist dress for a seventh grade dance and my plaid drill team kilt. Next to it is a stack of presto logs and milk jugs of water. In the original house plan, this room was to be a bomb shelter, and the power outage provisions echo the 1960's disaster preparedness. Shelves on the walls are filled with boxes of fabric and one labeled "George's Army Uniform." The bookcase includes Rebecca's entire set of Little House books by Laura Ingalls Wilder and a dozen tattered Little Golden Books. There are boxes of old Christmas decorations, including those handmade by my sisters and me in elementary school—pipe cleaner traces fallen off crushed egg carton sleighs. One of the barrels left over from our 1960 move holds old bedding, including the pilled blue blanket with worn satiny edging from my childhood bed and Jo Ann's faded red one with no edging at all. The family's entire past is in this room, safe from nuclear annihilation.

We start with the large cherry-stained dining table my father made that became Mama's craft table, where she flirted with quilting and silk painting. For months, and probably for years before my time here, she has been saying, "If that table were cleaned off, I could do projects and wrap gifts." What she wants is to be seventy again, or even eighty. What she wants is for the mess to be the only thing standing in the way of creativity. But now there is her sharply declining vision and cognition. The wishful thinking hurts my heart. I wonder how I can help, if I can help.

A few weeks ago, surreptitiously cleaning out drawers in my father's desk, I found a note in my mother's hand, sprinkled with shorthand I could only guess at: *Occasionally I seem to have a spurt of ambition to get things done and get back to some craft work. It seems that every day my energy is frittered away with not only the routine tasks that I've always done, but also taking care of George.* I rocked back in the office chair, blinking back tears. I recalled her inability in my childhood to sit with the family and read the Sunday newspaper, protesting that she didn't have time. Work always came first, and it was never done. I'm sure she learned at her hard-working mother's knee. Somehow I escaped the cycle.

I pick up a vintage cobalt blue glass Noxzema jar—a product that comes in plastic now—saved for a melted glass project she once dreamed of. I remove the lid. All vestige of the smell that would resurrect my adolescence when I used it to clean my acne-spotted face has been scrubbed out. I put it in the recycling bag, then take it back out and set it aside to keep.

"Do you want this?" she asks, holding up a small yellow ceramic Dutch shoe that had a florist's frog in it and held little bouquets in my childhood.

"Tell me about it," I say.

"It was a gift with flowers at the birth of one of you girls," she says simply. I wait for more, but that's all there is.

"I'm happy with the memory," I say.

"Put it in the box of things to ask Jo Ann and Rebecca about." I roll my eyes but dutifully put it in the box.

The silent butler crumb tray with no scraper, labeled "Made in Occupied Japan," with the Empire State building and other NYC tourist attractions etched on it, goes in a box to take to an antique store, joining other items that have been in the box for God knows how long and that will never make it to an antique store in her lifetime, nor off the table.

The table half cleaned off, Mama abruptly decides to get to the stuff on the floor in front of the shelves.

"Where did these come from?" I ask, holding up a paper bag of plastic champagne glasses."

"They're Rebecca's," Mama says. "Put them on the table to ask her about."

I send her a text message.

"She doesn't want them," I tell Mama, and put them in the empty Goodwill box.

There isn't anything else in front of the shelves, other than the large rolled up fake Navaho rug and one braided by my grandmother for our new family room. Michelle could have gotten to any of the fabric boxes.

It's lunchtime, and Mama is tired. A square foot of the table is bare. There are three things in the Goodwill box and a garbage bag of recyclables, which I take outside to the can immediately.

∾

Three weeks later, we resume the Great Table Clean-Off—which includes several new arrivals—so she can have room to wrap Christmas gifts in her fantasies. Mama and Michelle went to Goodwill, but the sack of Rebecca's plastic champagne glasses is still on the floor and at least two items from the throwaway box—that she told me not to throw away yet—are back on the table. What in God's name are we going to do with all this stuff when the time comes? I can't even go there.

While Mama rests from another unsuccessful attempt to clear the table, I go on a secret tear to clean off my father's old workbench, though a year ago I was told to leave it alone. The remains of my mother's long-abandoned crafting spill off the bench. I trash bottles of dried-up craft paint, solidified Drano, and hardened glue. I recycle baby food jars that used to hold homemade fabric dyes labeled dark blue, deep pink, light lavender, reminding me my mother used to have creative fun, used to be different. There are rocks, shells, and driftwood Mama and my father collected. Someday I will use them, along with the large collection from my childhood under the shed behind the carport, to make a memorial garden. I pick up a grocery produce bag containing dried roses from my wedding bouquet. A yellow sticky note, dated many years ago, reads: "Gretchen does not want these." They outlasted the marriage by twenty years. I cremate them and scatter the ashes in the garden.

A large canister takes up real estate on a corner of the bench. The note on top reads, "To be opened in 2025." I'm curious what set its contents apart from everything else in this time capsule house, but I leave it untouched.

❧

My deceit does not go unnoticed. I am summoned to the basement a few days later.

"I wish if you got it into your head to clean up you would ask for me to be here. It looks like you cleaned up the workbench."

"I threw out dried fabric dye and solidified Drano."

"Were there any good paints?"

"They are in the blue tub."

"I thought if I could get the table cleaned off, I might try some silk painting," she says.

A moment later, I have an idea. One of Rebecca's artist friends teaches silk painting in her home studio. Maybe Mama *could* do it again. I send my sisters a text. *What would you think about asking Sue to facilitate some silk painting time for the four of us at Christmas?* They respond immediately. *That's a great idea!* I send the teacher an email, pleased with myself for doing something proactive.

∽

A few days after our latest attempt to clear the table, she tells me why she can't get it cleaned off; or, if she did, the reason she can't do projects: there's a burned-out florescent bulb and she can't see. She needs to wrap a gift for her sister, and she berates me for not getting a bulb she hadn't asked me to get, so Stan the Handy Man could put it in today. There is still no room on the table to wrap gifts, but I drop everything and go downtown for a bulb, not wanting her to be angry with me all day. Stan installs it before he leaves.

"The light still doesn't come on," I tell Mama.

"Oh, it hasn't worked in years," Mama says.

33

December

Best Friends

I wake this morning ecstatic that it's my Olympia getaway day, and head upstairs.

"Did you put your sheets in the wash?" Mama says in response to my morning greeting.

"Oh, I forgot," I say.

She sighs, "We agreed you would do yours today so I could do mine tomorrow!"

"It's only nine o'clock. And how does mine not being in the wash yet affect you doing yours tomorrow?" I know she has no answer, and I don't expect one. Her obsession with the care and feeding of the septic tank is out of control. "Why don't you do yours today and I'll do mine another time."

"It's too late now," she sighs, turning back to the sink.

"Why is it too late? Michelle isn't even here yet to help."

"I want to go for a walk first thing!" Like I should have known that. Like she won't want to go for a walk first thing tomorrow too. I tell her I will strip her bed and start the wash.

I tell myself this is her bad day, that it has nothing to do with me, but my morning turns grumpy too. Letting other people's stuff be their stuff is a skill I continue to work on.

∿

Yoga, lunch, grocery shopping. My few hours of pretending I have a different life comes to an abrupt halt when Rebecca texts me between grocery stores wondering when I will be home. Mama's leg is "numb and tingling," though not, Mama reports, the severe cramps she gets occasionally. Fortunately Stan had been there after Michelle left and helped her. He'd stayed until Mama insisted she was okay, but as soon as he left she called Rebecca to come. Rebecca hung the "shut" sign on her shop door and dashed up the hill.

A few minutes later she texts again that Mama says she's better after elevating her leg, and is washing dishes. I rush through the rest of my shopping and when I get home an hour later she is still standing in the kitchen. She didn't take her afternoon rest and I'm not surprised when her leg starts hurting again at the dinner table.

"I wonder if I should call the on-call cardiologist," she says. "I don't want to have to go to the hospital in the middle of the night."

"Why do you think you would have to go to the hospital?" I ask.

"It might be a blood clot," she says.

"Ah," I say. I sure don't want to insist it's nothing; it could be a long night if she panics. We have all agreed she needs to avoid the hospital, but we have not yet been put to the test of muscling through her hysteria. I suggest she lie down and see if that helps. I help her get ready for bed and then massage her foot and put dryer-warmed towels on her leg until the cramp goes away.

When I check on her and tell her good night later, she tearily tells me she told Stan he was her best friend. Then she amends the statement, "Stan and Rebecca are the best friends I have."

"I'm glad they were here for you," I say. I turn up the baby monitor when I go to bed and listen to her breathe all night, afraid if I sleep I will miss her calling me.

34

January

Walking in the Dark

It's five thirty in the morning. I roll out of bed, feed Smudge, and brew coffee. Grabbing my laptop and mug, I head upstairs to my father's recliner that I have moved to a corner of the living room, creating a semiprivate space by the windows to wait for dawn to light the sky while Mama sleeps. It's the only time of day I feel alone in the house. I breathe differently during this hour, or two if I'm lucky.

The valley is filled with fog. The lights below are snuffed out, and it's very dark. I got through Christmas with visiting family, and I'm happy not to have to think about it again for months. The highlight of the long week was our studio time silk painting. I had to twist Mama's arm to get her to go, but she loved it. The teacher gave Jo Ann, Rebecca, and me gauzy blindfolds that let in just enough light to see some shadowy images of the materials we were working with, approximating Mama's vision. Her work was the best, but I gave myself extra credit for the idea to go. It was a glimmer of light piercing her dark world.

I travel back a year and a half to the life I walked out on. I rose early in North Carolina too, and pulled on clothes to walk to the historic cemetery to watch the sun come up over the old tombstones, then hurried home to shower and dress for work. My days then were productive, my work appreciated. I returned home each evening to my quiet home, prepared whatever I wanted for dinner, and ate in front of the fire with a good book, or on the patio under the dogwood tree, or on the deck with the birds, or on the sofa watching *Jeopardy*. Weekends were breaks from the workday routine: coffee shops and writing, gardening, creating, time with friends. My old life lurks in me like an old lover who is never coming back.

A successful day now is one in which I don't lose my patience with Mama and I manage to cook a meal she likes. We eat mostly in silence, neither of us being talkers and she increasingly unable to concentrate on both eating and conversing. I insist on opening the blinds behind her chair at dinner even when it's dark out; closed, the room feels as claustrophobic as my life here. Sometimes I fear I am losing my mind as quickly as Mama is disappearing into hers.

The sky is turning pink behind the mountain. I peer through the long feathery branches of the immense Douglas fir that block the view of the mountain, sky, and valley from nearly all the windows. They have become a metaphor for my life: all I can see is what is right in front of me. There is a hint of the future if I squint my eyes, but mostly I just have the stifling present. Having the branches trimmed up will be the first thing I do when Mama leaves us; when I will, finally, have an unobstructed view of the sunrise over the mountain as the sky—and my life—turns technicolor.

༄

I'm hopeful today will be a better day than yesterday, when Mama was more confused than usual, and unable to see anything. She went to bed at seven thirty, depressed and discouraged. I was worried. She seemed better this morning when I greeted her, but later falls apart.

I'm downstairs working when she calls me on the phone.

"I can't find my rice bags! I hate to bother you, but I have to lie down. And I can't find my bags," she says again. She sounds frantic, near tears.

I walk upstairs and find them in her bed.

"Here they are," I say. "You get in bed and I'll heat them for you."

She starts crying. Bags forgotten, I sit beside her on the bed and put my arm around her.

"I can't see or hear. I don't know what's going on," she sobs. "I was going to try to call Doris today, and I couldn't see to dial the number."

"You rest," I say, "and I'll help you call your sister when you get up."

"I can't relax until I call," she moans.

"I understand. But this doesn't seem like a very good time to call. I promise I'll help you later."

She accepts, finally, and is calm when I return with the warm bags, allowing me to tuck her in.

It's a rare expression of emotion that evokes more love and compassion in me than her complaining does. I wish I could reinterpret the complaining as her way of expressing fear and sadness and respond with compassion, but I seem incapable. I give her a kiss, wish her a good rest, and head for the bedroom door. She launches into Michelle before I can escape.

"I told Michelle to put some files I got out on the hearth, and she put them on the table next to it. She is so forgiving when I correct her, but I don't have the patience for her errors."

Grief piled on top of disappointment on top of grief on top of disappointment. I tell her I'm sorry and quietly pull the door shut behind me before she can say more.

❧

I take a walk of lucky timing later in the week in the feeble winter sun, the sky temporarily an impossibly blue canopy, wedged between grey sky and rain showers. The air is damp and fresh. A bird's nest downed by the weekend storm sits upright in the driveway. My soul takes a deep "yes" breath on this beautiful day, rising above the latest periodic slump of longing for my old life.

As I walk up this familiar hill in the seldom traveled opposite direction of town, I tumble into memory. "Go home the long way, Daddy," my sisters and I would plead when we pulled out of the Presbyterian church parking lot at noon each Sunday. We were loath to return to the humdrum of home and more hungry for a change of scenery than for Sunday dinner, which more likely than not was pot roast on a timer in the oven. Sometimes our father would oblige, and I would lean back in the seat and look out the window as we wound up and around the backside of the hill and arrived at our driveway fifteen minutes later than had we taken the direct, five-minute route. I wonder now if Mama shared our enthusiasm for the long route, or was she eager to be back in the haven of her kitchen taking care of her family?

I can't cajole Mama into cheerfulness when she is determined to be woeful, though I don't stop trying. Her depression is the third partner in a ménage à trois. I try to be happy for both of us, which makes a difference only to me.

I fear the map of old age she is drawing for me. I determine to take a different route home when my turn comes. For now, though, my task is to help her navigate her way home in the dark. I stumble over the terrain, and I rage, and I say I can't keep going. Then I regain my footing and I do keep going.

I repeat the mantra: *Please forgive me. I forgive you. I forgive myself. I love you.*

35

February

Mi Casa Es Su Casa

As my sojourn stretches beyond the planned year, I'm determined to stop draining my savings on a storage unit when I live in 3600 square feet of real estate. I've spent the past three months hauling carloads of boxes to the workshop over the carport after moving Rebecca's things from one side of the room to the other to make space. I've lined up moving help for Saturday for the five pieces of furniture left in the unit.

I made space on a shelf in the basement storage room by rearranging the contents, boxing up dozens of cheap picture frames to take to Goodwill without telling Mama; discarding nothing else. I moved long unused or never used miscellaneous items from a kitchen cabinet to the shelf I cleared, praying Mama won't get on her hands and knees and discover them gone. I use the partially emptied cabinet for some more of my own kitchen items.

I moved a bookcase to my bedroom so I could unpack my book boxes. The bookcase Rebecca painted for her use sat empty for five years until she cleared out the suite in preparation for my arrival and put it, inaccessible, behind an armchair in the guest room. The fallout comes two weeks later while I'm cooking dinner.

"What did you do with the bookcase in the guest room?" Mama asks.

"I moved it downstairs to put my books in. I didn't think it was being used."

"I was going to put shirts on it from the dresser and it wasn't there!"

Sticking to my vow of kindness, my word for the year, I apologize for not asking. I don't argue how ridiculous it is to use a bookcase as a clothes shelf, or suggest she pass on some clothes she doesn't wear. Closet shelves are filled with shoes in their original boxes and purses that once held tissues, moist towelettes, and Juicy Fruit gum. Drawers in three dressers hold sweaters and knit shirts, jewelry in white boxes, and her handkerchiefs with tatted edging and my father's monogrammed ones. Three double closets are crammed with custom-made and expensive—at least to her—department store dresses and coats from past decades. My mother had nothing as a child, other than hand-me-down clothes from neighbors and those her mother made from donated fabric or cut-down used dresses. I wonder if keeping these things is her proof that she rose above her upbringing.

I reach into my memory, searching for the mommy of my childhood, and all I find there is the closet. I follow the white gloves and clicking shoes across the shiny green tile floor of Miller's department store in Olympia. The purse comes off her arm to write a check for new curtains at Mottman's Home Goods to put in the basket that zipped up a line to cashiers in the balcony. I sit next to her dress at church and at the community concerts she sold season tickets for so she could take her family to every event.

I dig deeper. The dish gardens of moss and cones and tiny ceramic animals in aluminum pie plates she made with me. Her delight in the tiny bouquets of flowering weeds I brought her. Listening to my fumbling piano practice. Teaching my Sunday school class and leading my Girl Scout troop because she wanted those experiences for me. Drying my tears and dabbing stinging iodine on my scraped knees—turning the wound red and yellow—after letting me explore my world independently. I know her love for me is inestimable still. I open my heart to let it slip silently in.

Now, putting broccoli in the steamer and checking the salmon in the oven, I keep quiet through a long discourse on the history of the bookcase's unfinished-furniture origins and the store where it was purchased more than two decades ago that went out of business, but now there's a new store there and maybe they have another like it, and if I move her things in the kitchen she can't find them even if they are only moved six inches because she can't see, and she doesn't like venetian blinds but she needs something to block more light.

I listen without speaking, until she pushes my button: "I just need to move," she finishes. I explode like a jack-in-the-box. As irrationally as her harangue, I go off on Rebecca.

"If she would make time to organize her things in the workshop that she hasn't needed for eleven years, I wouldn't have to unpack boxes and move stuff into the house!" I rant. *And why could she use the bookcase and I can't?*

"She needs room to store her things too," she throws back. "You could sell your furniture and buy new when you have your own home." Not only my fury, but all my fears and doubts pop out with this final turn of the handle. My few possessions are all I have that is mine in this life that is not.

This is the only home I have. That she doesn't consider that floods me with renewed loss. And I don't know what I will do if she snatches away my dream of staying here; it's what keeps me going. My future terrifies me. That I have the earning power, as time out of the market and my age march on, to get a job that will pay me to live, let alone buy new furniture, seems ludicrous. I stuff it all back inside and shut the lid, cursing myself for letting the words and anger escape. I turn back to the stove and don't say another word.

❧

The fallout continues for the next forty-eight hours. Mama doesn't sleep, I don't sleep. Her stomach hurts, my heart hurts. Her back hurts. "Chair yoga did it," she says now, the private session I arranged for her six months ago after she said she'd always wanted to try it, then refused to do it again. My back hurts too, because I haven't been to yoga. She doesn't like what I cook. I don't like that there's no Valium on the menu.

She drafts her belated New Year's letter while I'm out: "Gretchen lives in the basement and cooks dinner for me," she writes. Later she edits it, deleting the part about me cooking her dinner.

❧

Three days later everything changes. My third grandson is born. I begin to spiral out into the world of this beautiful boy and his long future that I will be a part of. My sorrow at leaving my other two grandsons on the other side of the country lessens a bit.

My mother was sixty-three when Nicholas, her first grandchild, was born. I recently found a note in one of her collections in which she wrote of her envy of friends whose grandchildren were part of their lives, all four of her grandchildren growing to adulthood on the other side of the country. Having not been close to my grandmothers, even my mother's mother who lived nearby, I didn't understand her loss then—or my children's loss—until I left North Carolina. Now my heart breaks for her. As I grieve my distance from Max and Ethan, I rejoice in the arrival of this little one just eighty miles away. I am over the moon to be part of Elliot's life and he of mine. I hope he will lighten Mama's heart too.

As Mama spirals inward toward death, the threat of dragging me with her holds less power. I hold my grandson in my arms when he is less than twenty minutes old; this flesh of my flesh and bone of my bone. He opens his blue eyes and looks into mine and my world is in balance. This is home.

36

March

Building a Future

"I know why my abdomen has been bothering me," Mama tells me over dinner tonight. "It's the same problem I've had since the early nineties, when I went to the doctor with a bowel obstruction and he did a colonoscopy. I didn't hear from him until the follow-up visit a month later when he told me it was one of three things, one of which is cancerous. Or maybe it was five things, three of which were cancerous."

"Hmm," I say, which is becoming a standard response.

"I asked him why in the world he waited so long to tell me that. He brushed me off saying that if it was a cancer, it was very slow growing."

"Hmm."

"I was so angry at his attitude that I never went back."

"So you never found out which of the three things or five things it was?"

"No, but I know. It has been the problem ever since: a slow-growing cancer."

"Hmm."

"I'm not worried about it. I'm not going to do chemotherapy or anything." Indeed she seems gleeful—pleased perhaps with making the connection—and she doesn't need or want to talk about it. "I've had a good life. It's okay."

"Okay," I say, wondering how long it will be before it comes up again.

⌒

I lie in bed awake with an endless-loop tape running through my head of all the things I need to do, until I'm completely overwhelmed.

It's time for my own health exam, and I need a new doctor. I need to decide if I want to apply for social security. It's time to build my new garden in the meadow before it's too late to plant this year. I'm not writing as much as I want to. What if my car gives up for good? Minutia it's best not to obsess over in the middle of the night when everything feels like too much.

And then there's the big stuff. How and when will my mother's life end, what will happen between now and then, and can I hold out through that uncertainty? The paint on the fascia boards of the house is peeling, and if I tell Mama, she will say she doesn't want to put any more money into the place and we need to sell it before it needs anything else, and we'll be off and running on that again. When she is gone, can I keep this place up? Do I want the responsibility? Will I be able to afford to live here? Do I even want to live here? How will I afford to live anywhere else? The knee I had meniscus surgery on the year before I moved has been hurting, and my hip aches in bed. I'm aging too.

I finally sleep a little, and with my morning coffee I take action. I make a to-do list. It's not so onerous a list in the light of day. I leave off moving. I'm here as long as Mama is, and then the year it will take to clean out the house. At least that. I spend too much time trying again to figure out social security and mark it off my list without deciding what to do.

∾

Nicholas, Kristy, Max, and Ethan come to meet Elliot during their school spring break. Having them all here is a light in the gloom for both me and Mama, as she meets nearly two-year-old Ethan for the first time. It's only the third time I have seen him. They help me build boxes for my raised-bed garden in the meadow and Nicholas digs post holes. We play in the barn and walk in the woods. I wish they lived closer, or I had the resources to get them here for more visits. I long for Max and Ethan to visit me like my children visited their nana and papa here. But the era of children flying solo across the country, looked after by a flight attendant, ended on 9/11, as did the days of parents feeling comfortable allowing it. I will have to settle for seeing them once a year in North Carolina for now.

∾

I'm nearly despondent after they leave. I occupy myself building a fence around the three garden boxes with the water sprouts Stan the Handy Man pruned from the apple trees, old posts donated by the neighbor, and one-by-fours I find in the barn loft. Living in this house has made me a repurposing genius. I stop telling myself I can't build a gate and just do it. When I install it, I discover there's a gap under it on the sloping meadow. I need a solution before the rabbits find it. I fill the boxes with soil and plant peas and lettuce.

I learned from my father that all things can be accomplished. What he didn't pass on was how to do them, which peeves me now. But I'm figuring it out, one thing at a time—not his way, not the best way, but my way. Maybe he was wise to teach me "it can be done" rather than what Mama is still trying to impart: there's only her way. I find his measurement calculations for some long-ago project on a scrap of two-by-four, penciled in his familiar hand. He had to figure it out as he went too. I sit with the gate and come up with a "good enough" fix. I think he would be pleased that I got it done.

A few evenings later, as I'm cleaning up from dinner, I glance out the window. A rainbow arches across the valley, linking the two sides. It takes my breath away. All will be well.

37

May

Midnight in the ER

Mama hasn't felt well today. After dinner I ask her if she wants to walk up the driveway, thinking it might improve both her physical distress and her spirits. She holds my arm with one hand, her cane in the other. Halfway up the driveway she asks to see my garden, which she hasn't been in yet. I open the gate and help her through, careful with her on the uneven ground. I show her the squash plants in the first box, and the broccoli that may or may not amount to anything.

We are on our way to the peas and beans, which are doing well, when I step in a hole and lose my balance. Suddenly I'm pitching forward. Afraid I will take her with me, I yell, "Let go of me!" I desperately try to keep my feet under me as I hurtle toward the corner of the fence, falling into it, grabbing at the fence poles to keep from crashing through headfirst, scraping my fingers on the chicken wire. It takes me a few seconds to get up, glad for avoided catastrophe—like breaking my glasses, or bones. But when I turn around, Mama is on the ground face down. My heart stops. I stumble my way back to her and sink to the ground beside her.

Turning her over into my lap, I gasp. Her soft face is a bloody, already swollen and bruised mess. Her glasses are askew, clip-on sunglasses shattered. The neighbor across the driveway, cleaning up branches in his orchard, yells, "Should I call nine-one-one?"

"Yes! Yes!" I scream.

As he runs toward his house, I desperately try to call Rebecca on my cell phone with my left hand. I can't get my fingers to work. I try over and over. When I get through and she answers, I scream, "Get up here! Now!" I hear her running.

I can't get the phone disconnected. I'm shaking, my fingers are huge on the tiny buttons. Brad has brought a wet washcloth. I give up on the phone as I dab at Mama's face. It's good I couldn't disconnect. The phone is lying on the ground and Rebecca is able to hear what is happening and she keeps me from feeling so alone. "Damn train!" she rages. "Shit, shit, shit!" She says she thinks the ambulance coming from the fire station behind her apartment got across the tracks ahead of the train. She tells me she's turning around to go the several blocks to where she can cross the tracks on the viaduct. She doesn't know what happened, and she doesn't ask.

Mama calls out, "Goodbye, Gretchen, goodbye! I love you!"

"I love you," I tell her. "You're going to be okay." I say that, but I don't know. Is this the end?

I have never summoned an ambulance before, though I occasionally have nightmares of calling 911 and no one answers. Never have I been so happy to see anyone. Rebecca is there moments later. She must have been flying.

Mama is remarkably calm and has stopped expecting to see the bright light beckoning from the Great Elsewhere. She says she's okay, and that her legs feel fine. "I will still be able to walk," the most important thing. She tells me it's not my fault—which of course it is—and asks several times if I'm hurt.

The two EMTs are calm and efficient, and deftly defuse the fear with a bit of appropriate humor. They immediately see that her nose is broken and ascertain nothing else is. How can that possibly be? The orthopedist has told her she has "crappy bones." They bring the gurney into the garden, lift her onto it and into the ambulance. Telling Rebecca to ride with them, I race down to the house and grab the emergency suitcase I prepared just last night, eighteen months after the last time we went to the hospital and didn't know to have one. I wonder at the significance of the timing. It contains the packet of legal papers, warm socks, mango Burt's Bees lip balm—the creamiest flavor I've found. I grab Mama's bag with her ID and medical cards, and her medical journal. I throw in my phone cord and a book and Mama's favorite shawl.

Racing to the car, I blast up the driveway and stop behind the ambulance sitting at the road. Rebecca texts me they are pausing to splint Mama's arm because she is complaining of pain. As I wait, drumming my fingers on the steering wheel, taking deep breaths to stay calm, I vaguely wonder how much ambulance transport costs. Nothing, it turns out. Medicare and supplemental insurance—paid by my father's retirement benefit—covers every penny of every health crisis and routine doctor and specialist visit except for dental cleanings and having her toenails cut by the podiatrist.

Finally on the move again, I follow them across town: no speeding, no sirens, no life-threatening injuries. I can see Mama's face through the back window: her bruised and swelling face looks terrible, but she's alert. They sit her up a bit and I watch her conversing with the EMT. I start breathing again, but I feel sick for her. I cry most of the way across town to the hospital.

Arriving by ambulance gives us a Pass the Waiting Room Free card. They ask only once what meds she is on, rather than every time a new person comes into the room. Last time I had only been living here three months and had to depend on Rebecca to tell them. This time I know all the over-the-counter meds and not only the one prescription she takes and the one she recently stopped taking, but how to pronounce them. I know what her weight and blood pressure were at the last ten doctor visits, thanks to the journal that travels with us. But they know too. All her records from both hospital and doctor visits are now in the computer. Digital progress.

X-rays and a CT scan are done. Unlike last time, Rebecca and I are in the room beside her or behind the screen the whole time. We are learning to navigate this journey. Nothing is amiss other than an "uncomplicated" broken nose. Nothing is uncomplicated in Mama's world, though, and I expect it will become a major issue. There is no concussion, no bleeding on the brain. I wonder if it would have been a different story had she not finally stopped taking the blood thinner, months after the cardiologist ordered its discontinuation in part for the possibility of an event like this.

The staff is impressed with Mama's support system. A nurse in Mickey Mouse scrubs tells us of the appalling number of elderly people in real or imagined crisis who come through the ER alone. I'm glad again I am here, though she wouldn't have fallen if she hadn't trusted me to keep her safe.

We are sent home at three thirty in the morning with a new splint and sling for the arm a second X-ray confirms nothing is wrong with, and a prescription for Tylenol with codeine.

∾

Rebecca spends the next two nights in the guest room, getting up in the night when Mama calls for help to the bathroom, or in a panic because she can't breathe deeply, or is in pain. She won't take the

Tylenol. I turn off the monitor and try to sleep so I can cope with the days. I hear every movement through the heat vents all night. In a stroke of bad luck, Michelle is on a pre-scheduled vacation.

"I'm so tired," Rebecca says when she arrives at the house for night three.

"It's not right," I say. "At least I can take a nap; you have to work! She has to take the Tylenol."

I help Mama get to bed while Rebecca has a second glass of wine. I heat her rice bags and deliver them with a Tylenol tablet and glass of water.

"What's that?" Mama asks.

"It's Tylenol," I say, holding my breath, waiting for the push back.

"Regular or extra-strength?"

Should I lie? Definitely. But I don't. "It's Tylenol with codeine, prescribed by the doctor."

"I don't like to take medication," she says. My Therapeutic Lie skills need improvement.

"I know you don't. But you need to get better sleep. And Rebecca and I aren't sleeping either. We can't take care of you if we don't sleep."

She considers that. Perhaps self-care doesn't persuade her, but the chance to take care of her daughters gives her pause. "Okay," she says finally.

She sleeps. I sleep. Rebecca gets up several times to check on her. I can't fix Rebecca.

"I can take it from here," I tell her when she leaves for work the next morning, looking exhausted.

"Are you sure?" she asks.

I laugh, sort of. "No," I say, "but let's see how it goes."

I'm on my own. I move upstairs to sleep to be closer to Mama. I give the days to her and her needs, and don't lament that I canceled first one haircut appointment and then the rescheduled one, and a dentist appointment, and I will be at the ENT with her tomorrow rather than at yoga. I haven't left the property in days except to go to the grocery store. I'm struggling with the possibility I will have to give up a long-scheduled, five-day respite retreat. I am aware this is but a small window into what so many other caregivers do day in and day out, and I try to suck it up.

◞◟

The sixth day after the fall, Mama gets herself up for breakfast.

"Wow!" I say, when she comes into the kitchen. "You're dressed! And the swelling is way down!" I'd noticed it was receding as the brilliant purple and blue on her face turned yellow, but the improvement this morning is startling.

"I thought I would feel better if I got out of bed," she says.

"And do you?"

"Yes," she says. "I think so."

Michelle is returning tomorrow too. I nearly cry with relief.

Rebecca and I both take her to a prescheduled doctor's appointment with another new provider after Lisa, whom we all loved, moved to Idaho. The visit was to be about her ongoing abdominal complaints, which she hasn't mentioned since the accident. The doctor is surprised at her quick recovery. I'm not. In spite of her complaining nature, she is resilient.

Friends and family continue to reassure me that the accident wasn't my fault. Mama theorizes that she pulled me off balance, and she doesn't blame me. I'm grateful for their words, but I know I bear responsibility, if not fault.

◞◟

With Michelle here in the mornings, Mama improves enough to be alone in the afternoons. Rebecca spends nights at the house and I go on my planned retreat to the beautiful home of a vacationing friend on the edge of Puget Sound's Sinclair Inlet. I watch the ferries and the eagles; commune with her cat; sit on the deck in the sun; and read, write, and sleep.

38

May

Forever Young

After Mama goes to bed tonight, I get Simon & Garfunkel's *Parsley, Sage, Rosemary and Thyme* album out of the metal box of vinyl records I've hung onto and put it on the old stereo console in the living room. The cabinet, with its 8-track player, sits there looking like an ordinary piece of 1960s modern furniture, but it smells of childhood closed up under the hinged lid, like a time capsule holding my youth in. I'm stunned for a moment that those evenings we "sang along with Mitch" are gone, that my sisters aren't here, that my father will never be here again, that soon my mother won't be. I listen to the whole album: "Feelin' Groovy," "Sounds of Silence," the seven o'clock news headlines layered over "Silent Night."

Several years ago, I discovered an army footlocker—the large flat-topped metal boxes designed by the military to fit under a soldier's bunk to hold literally everything they were allowed to carry with them—in the outdoor storage shed and pried open the lid. I was stunned to find it held five hundred letters written by my father to my mother during WWII and ninety-nine surviving letters she wrote to him. I brought them into the house and put them in an airtight plastic container on a shelf in the basement where they sat forgotten until I moved back home. I finally pulled them out over the winter and began reading them.

First Mama didn't want me to read them to her. "I only kept them because I thought if I had children they might want to read them after I was gone," she said. I messed up her plan and found them before she died. Then she changed her mind. "I would like you to read the letters to me," she said out of the blue one day. I was glad, thinking she could clear up some mysteries. But when I ask her for back story to my father's one-sided conversations, she usually says, "I have no idea." They were two people eking out a love story in circumstances I can't imagine. What is left are these letters written seventy years ago by a young man, layered with the sketchy memory of an ancient woman. And my questions that will never be answered.

I open the notebook of letters that I have put in archival sleeves and start reading while "Flowers Never Bend with the Rainfall" plays on the stereo. My father spent the first months of his nearly four years of war duty at New York University in officer training and a meteorology course. The cadets were about to get their first leave and he would see his love for the first time in four long months, over which he wrote sixty letters to her.

> *March 14, 1943*
>
> *Dearest—*
>
> *What kind of thoughts do you think go through a fellow's head when he's all alone in New York and when he doesn't like the place? They are many and varied, I assure you. The song on the radio is "Johnny Doughboy Found a Rose in Ireland." Why do they have to play that tonight? The memories are so strong and I'm thinking of you so hard tonight.*
>
> *This afternoon, I saw a US recruiting service station wagon*

parked. When this mess is over, I'm going to buy one of those. I'm going to fill it with camping equipment. I'm going to marry you. I'm going to take six months to do those things I've always dreamed of. We're going out west. We're going to see every bit of the country from Mexico to Canada. With you I'm going to sit on some peak and fill my eyes with thousands of acres of land and trees and mountains and sky. And I'm going to fill my arms with the girl I love and I'm going to forget the years in the army fighting a war that nobody wanted.

    Then a uniform approaches with bars on it. I have to salute. I'm not in a steep-walled valley. It's only the canyon that is Fifth Avenue. I know anyone who looked closely would have seen me muttering; and if he could have heard, it wouldn't have been nice.

    George

As I read these letters to my mother, I wonder, *Did she think she would always be young?* Now she doesn't go out the front door alone. The occupational therapist recommends she not go down the interior stairs alone either, because of a risk of falling. But she does not heed his "advice." She chooses not to go outside without help, but no one is going to *tell* her what to stop doing. Did she ever consider in 1943 that her life would come to this?

When I was a child, I thought in some unreachable depths of my soul the halcyon days at my first home by the bay in Olympia would never end and nothing bad would ever happen. But the days did end, when I was eight, and we moved thirty miles down I-5, a move that separated childhood from the rest of my life. A president was assassinated, my school bus slid down an embankment, my sister left home, my best friend moved away, boys ignored me, headlines screamed death tolls in Vietnam in 72-point font—"Hey, hey, LBJ; how many kids did you kill today?" I grew up.

Did I think my children would never leave home, that I wouldn't always be the young mother they loved more than anything or anyone? Wouldn't I always be sitting on the sidelines cheering for their soccer teams? I would never divorce; never leave my home and my friends.

And now do I think I will always be able to haul bricks and fifty-pound bags of paver sand, dig in the garden, hike in the mountains, drive a car? I live with my ninety-seven-year-old mother. With her aging in my face every day, I don't have the luxury of ignoring the fact that someday I won't go out the front door without help.

My mother's life rushes through me like a river overflowing its banks as I read her youthful words. I feel her loneliness and fear through those long years apart, letters their only connection. Yet they are devoid of any real information that would have been neatly cut out of his by the censor, hers putting on a happy face for him as directed by the United States government.

The voices on the album sing on and suddenly I am my mother, embodying her sorrow. Her love is once more beyond her reach. Hearing the letters makes her sad. For fleeting moments, she says, she thinks George is just away again; that as before, he will come home soon. But she knows he isn't ever coming back.

It is a thin line between joy and sorrow. When do we begin realizing that we *will* bend and life *will* end?

39

June

Mother Load

"Gretchen? Gretchen!" It's one o'clock in the morning. I groan and drag myself upstairs. She's trying to fix her pillows, she's not comfortable. She needs an extra-strength Tylenol. The regular one she took—though I encouraged her to take the stronger one—isn't doing the trick. It takes her five minutes to decide she does not want the humidifier on. I return to bed and can't get back to sleep.

Sometime after dawn I finally sleep briefly, until Smudge starts walking on me and whining for breakfast at six o'clock. I feed her and go back to bed. A few minutes later, the plaintive "Gretchen?" comes over the monitor again. I trudge up the stairs. "Would you take my temperature?" she says. "I think I have a fever."

"The damn room is a hundred and eight degrees, who wouldn't be hot?" I snap, too tired to be patient. I know she hates it when I swear, though she never says anything.

"Well, it wasn't so hot when I thought I had a fever, but I didn't want to bother you then."

"You felt feverish, so you closed the window and turned the heat up?" I don't expect a response. I take her temperature and report that it's 97.5.

"That's normal for me," she says, like she hasn't told me that a million times. "I had two good BMs in the night, so my stomach feels good now."

"Glad to hear it," I say.

∽

The next day I go to a meeting in Seattle for my very part-time job. Stan the Handy Man spends the day with Mama. It's heavenly to get away, though I'm sad I can't see Elliot; they have house guests. I need a baby fix and I'm sorry I didn't ask for just ten minutes.

As we eat dinner after my return, I ask Mama if she enjoyed the day. "It was a beautiful day," she says. "If I could hire Stan one full day a week I wouldn't need Michelle." I nearly spit out my mouthful of food. Michelle comes four mornings a week, the only reason I'm still functioning.

"I don't think you realize all Michelle does for you," I say when I recover.

"Well, I could hire you to do what she does, but I don't think you could tolerate it."

"You're right. Not going to happen. I came here to be your daughter and companion, not your employee." She has no idea what I do for her either.

∽

After dinner, I walk up the driveway to my garden. I've barely been there since the fall. PTSD. I repair the fence in two places where I fell into it. I pocket a piece of Mama's shattered clip-on sunglasses. Because of her swollen nose, she was unable to wear her glasses or clip-ons and had to depend on her visor to shade her eyes. She will never wear her glasses again, and they sit useless alongside the reading glasses we got that she has never used. I wonder if she's secretly relieved to give up the strenuous task of trying to continue to read the newspaper, no longer reminded of yet another loss.

I check the progress of the broccoli and beans, plant more lettuce and chard, and thin what's come up. Though she will occasionally peer through the fence into my garden, a few steps from the driveway, Mama never goes through the gate again, declining all my offers and reassurances.

I hope she soon will get back to the tiny bit of flower bed by the front door she still tends, leaving the rest in Stan's hands, trusting he has learned her lessons, what is weed and what is not. She has flowers to plant and weeds to pull, and that will help her heal. Though I haven't beaten myself up for her fall, if she is unable to enjoy her own patch of dirt again, I may find my way to guilt after all.

year three

40

July

Cheerleader Mom

I'm doing the dishes when Mama comes into the kitchen from the bathroom. She wants to know what the "two white squares" are in the yard below the second story bathroom window. I haven't told her yet I'm making a shade garden there, an area that has always been a wasteland. I curse myself for leaving in her sight line the only evidence she could see. A year ago she told me I was welcome to work on that space, challenging me, perhaps, to spin straw into gold. She's forgotten she sparked the idea. I tell her they are bags of soil and she is so mad I'm afraid she will stop breathing.

"George tried to do something there, and grass won't grow," she snaps.

"I'm not growing grass," I say, mystified by her anger.

"Nothing will grow but moss. I've tried to grow ferns there."

"And ferns *are* growing there."

"I don't want you to do anything there! It's a waste of money and time."

"I used my money," I lie.

"It's *all* my money."

"No, I'm using *my* money," I repeat.

"You mean from your bank account?"

"Yes," I say, diving deeper into the deception. She thinks I don't have any money, having plunged deeply into her own story that I'm completely dependent on her and came to live with her because I couldn't take care of myself.

"Well," she says, drawing out the word, "if you want to waste your money that's your business! But next time tell me before you start something."

"I will do no such thing. You will sap all the joy out of the project, like you just did. If I had listened to all the naysayers in my life, including the one in my head, I would not have done lots of things that turned out great. Maybe it won't work, I've had failures too, but I need to try. I'm an adult, and I need to do some one thing my way!"

My filters have left the building. She doesn't speak. My shoulders slump. I've done it again: she's going to collapse into tears. But she doesn't.

"I'm proud of you," she says finally. "You are like me, thinking I couldn't speak in public, but I did it anyway."

The Peace Ribbon Project, back in the mid-eighties when I was preoccupied with raising two small children in our new home in Mississippi, was conceived as a protest against nuclear war, the idea being to wrap the Pentagon with a mile of banner, its tied-together sections created by people around the country on the theme, "What I would hate to lose in a nuclear war." When Washington's state coordinator dropped the ball, my mother unofficially stepped in, collected banners, and delivered them to Washington, DC, for the event, which ended up with not one, but eighteen miles of "ribbon." When she returned home, she took her experience on the road, speaking to church and civic groups in the area, powering through her reticence to speak before crowds.

"Yep," I say, letting out my breath, "I learned it from your example. And I was proud of you too."

It's a tiny breakthrough.

❧

I clean out the little chalet barn my father built for our horse Scout: a roll of barbed wire; the cage Rebecca's guinea pigs, Pig One and Pig Two, lived in; another cage that was home to my father's rescued baby flying squirrel, "Lil Guy," that traveled in his shirt pocket until he released it back to the wild. I rake through the debris on the dirt floor—decomposed leaves, mouse-chewed cardboard, a petrified mouse—and throw it out the door into the woods, earth to earth. In the bottom of the manger, under tomato cages and driftwood and a box of horseshoes, is the lead rope for Scout's halter. I hold it in my hand for several moments, lost in nostalgia, then hang it over the rusted Maxwell House coffee can nailed to a timber where the bridle hung forty-five years ago.

I climb the attached ladder into the hay loft—the floor spackled now with bat guano—and remember when my neighbor Barbara and I tried to overnight here when we were in fifth and sixth grades, but got scared and went back to the house; and when my high school boyfriend Marc and I chastely trysted here. I recall the chores: grabbing a bale of hay with hooks, dragging it to the edge, pushing it over to be pulled apart and put in the manger along with a coffee can of oats; mucking the stall and putting down fresh straw; combing Scout's coat with the curry comb. I'm amazed I did all that, realizing my strength has history. I think about my father's farming boyhood and see how he didn't leave his childhood behind, but brought it here to this place and taught his daughters self-reliance by his quiet example. He was our silent cheerleader.

When I find two mouse-chewed fingers of his work glove, I sink down in the doorway and sob. I want time back.

I move outside the barn and sit on a section of log I rolled there for a bench, leaning my head back against the wall. It's time to return to the house to get Mama ready to go a memorial service, but I take a few more moments in the sun. Mama's friends, all younger than she, are leaving this world. She is ready to move on too, but her body tenaciously clings on. *When will it be her turn?* I ask the Universe, wondering how it feels to be left behind.

The answer comes whispering through the tall firs: *She is going to stick around until you learn to love and accept her for who she has been, in all her imperfection, and for who she is now, still imperfect. Only then, will you be able to be at peace with her now and with your-self when she is gone.*

I bolt upright. I know it's my head telling me what I already know, but I have yet to learn to live into it.

I have to accept her: blind, deaf, insecure, controlling, fearful, depressed, pessimistic. And brave. I need to release her from the person I wish she were: funny, grace-filled, happy, appreciative. I need to let go of the relationship I wish we had: best friends, confidantes, and champions of each other. One more chance to find that relationship may be why I came to live with her. But this is the mother I was given, and I am proof that she has always been enough.

I'm startled at the clarity. I've learned a lot in two years, but this final most important lesson of acceptance is elusive. It's an acceptance in need of constant vigilance and repair, not a place to arrive and relax into. I long to be able to carry this responsibility with grace and ease and compassion, but perhaps that's not to be either. Maybe that's the second most important lesson, to accept myself for who I am: a flawed human, like all humans, doing the best I can. And I am enough.

Those who are not walking this walk tell me I am so lucky to have a parent still with me and someday I will be so glad I did this. They probably had a cheerleader mom, or were fantasizing that they would have, had she lived longer. I want to tell them they are full of shit, but I don't. We all have our burdens.

I've been here 730 days, and I still have much to learn, and no idea how much time I have.

41

October

Baby Love

When school started after Labor Day, and Wynne—a new kindergarten teacher—began her first job, Rebecca added an overnight on the hill to her schedule, and I added two days a week with Elliot to my caregiving role. It helped them reduce infant care costs and gave me precious time with him. After a month, I've got the routine down. On Monday mornings, I leave my warm bed at five o'clock and dress quickly. Smudge doesn't mind missing her morning scratch as long as I feed her. I nuzzle her goodbye and go upstairs. Quietly pushing open Mama's bedroom door, I step into the warm-mist humidifier sauna that is her sanctum at night and listen for her breathing. Hearing the snuffle that accompanies every fourth or fifth silent intake and exhalation, I whisper an unheard, "See you tomorrow" and back out of the room, pulling the door shut. At the front door, I pick up my tiny suitcase—the one my father gave my mother in 1943, that I found in a high cabinet—and step out into the crisp autumn air, locking the door behind me.

I descend the hill into fog and drive to my favorite of the many espresso kiosks downtown to pick up my sixteen-ounce low-fat, half-caff, extra hot latte when they open at five thirty. The barista knows my order by now and starts making it when she sees me pull into the lot. I'm ascending the interstate ramp by five forty.

I roll along through the fog with the trucks, sipping my latte and listening to my recorded book. Across the prairie, the sky begins to lighten subtly. A few weeks ago the sun rose across the ground fog behind Mt. Rainier here, but now it's mostly dark, and the fog reaches into the tops of the tall, ghostly firs. Traffic picks up in Tacoma and doesn't let up until I exit I-5 an hour later on the outskirts of Seattle, switching to SR 509 where I can breathe again. I come over the rise of the drawbridge across the ship canal to the view of the Emerald City as the rising sun bounces off the glass-sided skyscrapers. The SR 99 viaduct skirts Puget Sound with the Olympic Mountains beyond as the ferries and freighters chug across the sparkling water.

I arrive at Emma and Wynne's apartment by eight, early morning traffic making the trip an hour longer than it should be. Elliot is sitting on the quilt I made for him surrounded by toys. He looks up when the front door opens. His eight-month-old face breaks into the most amazing smile. I put my suitcase down and swoop him up. He belly laughs. His delight in seeing me is remedy to my mother's constant frustration with me, with her bowels, with her diminished life, and with my own feeling that I've failed her and maybe myself.

Emma sits with her breakfast and we chat. I play with Elliot while she showers and dresses; then it's the two of us for the day. I clean up the kitchen and work on a task for my small job or on a writing project while he takes his morning nap. We play, eat, walk to the library or the swings or nowhere in particular; eat, nap, play.

In the evening, I enjoy dinner and time with my girls, grateful for their youthful energy that replenishes mine. Tuesday morning I'm there to play when Elliot gets up. When school is out I take him to Wynne's classroom two blocks away and hit the interstate traffic again for the trip home.

∽

Mama looks up from her recliner tonight when I unlock the front door and walk in, calling out, as always, "Is that Gretchen?" She is happy to see me. I reverse my Monday morning steps, going downstairs, dropping off my suitcase, feeding Smudge. I return to the kitchen to fix dinner, which Mama—already over being glad I'm back—criticizes as she tells me about her chronic constipation and dissatisfaction with her days, especially over Michelle, while I was away. While she whines, I wine.

She resumes her complaints as I clean up after dinner. I guess it was a bad day, and who knows why? Certainly not Mama.

I say good night and turn toward my sanctuary for the night, where only Smudge complains, and I can ignore her. "Thank you for all your patience," Mama says to my back. I stop in my tracks, then turn and tell her I'm sorry I don't have more. "Well, that's understandable," she says. "You're remarkable."

"Thank you," I say. "You are remarkable too." And I mean it.

42

January

Care Partner Crisis

Mama continued to be more confused through December, to sleep poorly, to complain of this or that malady—made up and not—as I sank into my annual holiday slump. Maybe Christmas is a hard holiday for her too. If we ever really talked, I would know the ways we are more the same than different.

After the holidays, I take a break to the Whidbey Island home of vacationing friends, watching the snowy Olympic Mountains break through the clouds across Puget Sound. I walk and play with my friends' corgi, read, write, chop wood, sleep, prepare simple meals, watch the sun set over the mountains, sit by the wood stove, soak in the hot tub under the stars, and sleep some more. I start breathing again. If nothing else, I have mastered self-care.

While I'm away, Rebecca sends reports of the action at home: downtown Centralia floods in an epic rainfall, Mama ramps up her talk of looking for a new paid caregiver, a squirrel gets in a transformer box and knocks out the power at the house. And the freezer door is left unlatched for an undetermined number of hours, tantamount to Fort Knox being plundered with the loss of Mama's soup supply and my precious leftover refried beans, homemade risotto, and chicken pie filling for meals when I can't bear to think about what to have for dinner. Rebecca shoulders it all, earning a new jewel in her crown and a break herself. When I return, she crosses the country for her annual markets to buy product for her shop, with no way to get back for a crisis. And it's coming.

∽

My first morning home, rested and ready to keep going, I head for my day in Olympia. As I drink coffee and write my weekly blog post, my phone rings. It's Michelle, in tears. She and Mama have had an altercation. Mama "invited" her to leave employment, and she accepted. "I wanted to be with her until the end," Michelle says through her tears, "but I can't do it anymore. I love her, but she is so mean to me. I have to take care of myself." I listen to her story, fighting back my own tears of rage and dread.

I'm furious with Mama. I haven't engaged with her stories about Michelle's alleged shortcomings—ones Michelle occasionally has also told me with a laugh—because Mama wants to be in charge of her employees and I have tried to let her, within reason. When she told me she got upset with Michelle for tossing her ponytail and hitting her in the eye and Michelle told me she hadn't done that, I just said I was sorry. When Michelle told me Mama accused her of not following directions when she drove her to a friend's house, taking a different route, I told Michelle I was sorry. I have heard daily complaints from Mama, but didn't realize she was voicing them all to Michelle. Maybe I should have been more involved.

I decide not to return home early to deal with the crisis. I need meditative yoga to get past my furor, letting Mama stew alone for a while in the mess she has made.

Hours after Michelle's call, I am calm and determined to remain so when I get home. I wait for Mama to bring it up.

"Did Michelle call you?" she asks finally as I'm cleaning up the kitchen—left undone in Michelle's abrupt departure—so I can start dinner.

"She did," I say.

"I didn't fire her!" she says adamantly.

"What happened?" I ask calmly.

I listen to her elaborate and incongruous storytelling, a recounting that differs significantly from Michelle's, holding none of Mama's ire and irrationality and placing all the blame on Michelle's alleged bad mood. "Michelle lost her temper when I asked her what time it was," she says.

She doesn't tell me the bit about sniping at Michelle for glancing up at the clock rather than looking at the new watch she bought for herself at Mama's insistence, so she could tell her how long it took to walk a lap at the mall. I know when I engage in her dementia what I mean to be conversation always ends with nothing resolved and both of us feeling bad, and for once I wait. When she finishes, I simply say, "The bottom line is you are without a caregiver."

"I guess that's what you're here for, Gretchen. I pay your room and board, and your utilities. Could you afford that if you weren't living with me?"

I don't crack, calmly reiterating my boundaries.

"Well, I just need to move then," she says. Several times in the coming months I will wonder if this was the moment I should have told her we would start looking for placement.

Rebecca is gone. I curse the bad luck, which may have been

Mama's plan: divide and conquer. I call the agency the next day and ask for a new caregiver on a trial basis. She has a three-day honeymoon before she falls short of Mama's standards: she couldn't find the pea soup recipe and didn't know how to use the VitaMix; and they didn't get all the errands done, there being too many on Mama's list to fit the available time. There's another one waiting in the wings. The choice will be Mama's, and it may take a while. No one will please her, at least not for long. She can't bear to need help.

I haven't seen David in months. I make an appointment, then cry through it while he tells me yet again this is hard work and I'm doing fine. It doesn't feel fine.

43

April

Bookends

It's a rare warm early spring day. We've limped along through a series of unsatisfactory caregivers since January. Today it's just the two of us, and I ask Mama if she would like to try to walk in the woods. She doesn't think she can, her standard response when I suggest it. I persuade her to try to go a little way. I help her bundle into her oversized warm jacket—big enough to wear her wool sweater under—hat, scarf, and gloves, and we set out up the driveway and into the forest.

I walk beside her where the trail is wide enough, or slightly behind where it's not, holding her hand, moving slowly. So much has changed since we first walked here together nearly three years ago, with me just following behind her. Now she leans on her cane. I am her eyes, telling her when she needs to step over a root or where there is a change in the terrain.

She asks me if I see this plant or that. I have to ask her what they look like because I have no idea. I wish I had asked her to teach me over all these years, instead of being impatient of her with her camera. It feels like too little too late now. I have wanted her to ask me about my life, but I have never asked her about hers.

"I never thought I would be here again," she says as we walk, wonder edging her voice. "Thank you, dear Gretchen." I have done something right, and my heart swells.

∽

A few days after our walk, I'm starting dinner when Mama gets up from her nap and comes into the kitchen. Meals have been quick and easy for several days, so I'm going all out with pork tenderloin, chard, roasted parsnips, sautéed apples. I'm happy to be taking the time to prepare a mindful meal.

"Did you rest well?" I ask.

"I'm not paying anyone else who isn't a CNA," she says.

"What do you think you need that a CNA can provide?" I ask, jumping into the rabbit hole with her.

"She can't make soup and she doesn't wash her hands," she says of the newest candidate.

"I'm sure she washes her hands," I say, ignoring the soup complaint, "but that has nothing to do with being a CNA. Aides who work for an agency are trained in basic caregiving skills and personal hygiene. Certified Nursing Assistants are trained to help the client bathe, go to the bathroom, dress, eat, and monitor medications. You don't need that kind of care right now. The rest is personality, not training. I'm not crazy about her either," I add in a conciliatory tone. "Someone else is coming on Monday; maybe we will like her better."

"I'm not paying for a CNA if I'm not getting a CNA."

"You aren't paying the CNA rate," I say, edging into exasperation.

"If they can't provide a CNA, I want to advertise in the paper for one."

"Dinner will be ready in forty-five minutes," I say, turning back to the cutting board.

I don't remind her she has had two CNAs and she didn't like either of them, or suggest someone she finds in the paper isn't vetted. We both miss Michelle, as I knew we would. Mama admitted regretfully last week that she hadn't appreciated what she had. That bridge has burned. It's an agency policy that if a placement ends on bad terms, the agency does not allow reemployment, for the protection of the employee.

We sit down to dinner, and Mama says she can't eat what I have prepared.

The next day, she tells Rebecca that the aide told her she doesn't need a CNA—forgetting it was I who told her—and she wants to know why she's paying for a CNA when she doesn't need one. "Gretchen is losing her memory," she adds. "It's worse than mine."

∽

Monday morning I'm in my car at five thirty, heading to Seattle for my days with Elliot, fourteen months old now. Two-and-a-half hours later, I have traversed the interstate divide between the oldest and the youngest members of the family. These bookends of my life are wells of neediness and fountains of determination to be impossibly self-reliant.

Emma and Wynne have moved from their apartment, with its long flight of cement steps down to the sidewalk along a busy street, to a tiny hundred-year-old rental house with a picket-fenced yard next to a Buddhist monastery. I carry a sobbing Elliot to the end of the sidewalk to wave goodbye to his mommy over the fence as she pulls out of the driveway. All will be well in a few minutes, but right now I'm a lousy substitute. A man is in the grassy parking strip under the trees in front of the monastery as he is each Monday morning. His bicycle and helmet lie on the ground beside him. He flows through the slow, rhythmic movements of tai chi as Elliot watches, gulping air as he calms himself from the betrayal of being left. He loosens his grip on my neck as his livid face morphs to sad, then curious, then delighted in a flash.

He squirms to be put down. He is still in his footed dinosaur pajamas, but I lower him to the ground and unlatch the gate. I do a half sun salutation. Elliot puts his hands on the ground beside me in downward facing dog, then stands up and toddles down the sidewalk toward the man. He stops and does another down dog while I watch from the gate.

The man turns his head and smiles at Elliot, then waves. Elliot puts his palms on the sidewalk again in one more perfect pose, then stands up laughing. The man does his own down dog in the grass—not something I have observed him doing in his usual practice—then stands up and chuckles, his eyes twinkling at Elliot. Elliot claps his hands in appreciation. The man puts his hands together in *anjali mudra*—prayer position—and bows slightly. *Namaste: the light within me honors the light within you.*

Each morning when I greet Mama with a cheery "Good morning!" she tells me all that is wrong with the day already. Some mornings I let her be, sometimes I ask her to tell me one good thing, guiding her to it:

"Did you get out of bed unassisted?"

"Yes, but I should have gotten up earlier. I thought I would just lie back down and 'take my exercises,' but I went back to sleep."

"I'm glad you were able to get up by yourself. I'm glad you can still exercise!"

My attempts at encouragement are met with silence.

It's hard to give up wanting her to be someone she is not, but I won't be drawn into her chronic dissatisfaction. I'm learning to let go of all that is no more in my life and to stop wanting something other than what I have. To be satisfied with this smiling toddler who interrupted morning meditation on this grass under these trees, and so quickly forgot his trauma. To be satisfied with knowing I am the reason Mama can still get out of bed in her own home in the morning. To tell myself that when she tells friends, "My children won't let me move," that maybe it's her version of gratitude. As I learned to be content that I was a good enough mother, I am learning to be content that I am a good enough daughter, and maybe I am more than a good enough grandmother.

44

June

The Trunk

I open the creaky door to the storage room tonight to return an empty canning jar to the shelf on my way to bed, and a buried trunk suddenly catches my attention. Mama stashes plastic cleaner's bags, flat rate post office boxes, and bubble wrap on top of it. A half sheet of typing paper taped to the side says, "Mom's things"—her mother's. I assumed that was what is in it and have not paid it much attention.

I am crazy to find the rest of the letters my mother wrote to my father, if they still exist. It's unlikely—not even possible really—that they are here, but what is under that lid? Is it really merely knick-knacks from my grandmother's tiny apartment? I need to know. I clear the top and pull the metal trunk out from under the cabinet above, revealing a pill bug and dried centipede graveyard. I sit down on the painted cement floor and flip open the stiff latches, pushing up the heavy lid.

On top of the tray, in a plastic bag, is the hearth rug Jo Ann crocheted as a gift to my parents decades ago, with a note taped to it in Jo Ann's perfect handwriting: *"Give this away. I do not want it."* Like everything else that has outlived its usefulness, it was stashed in this room after Mama failed in her attempt to give it back to Jo Ann. I put the bag on the floor and glance through a pile of papers: newspaper clippings, magazine articles, the extra copies of service bulletins and invitations to the celebration of my marriage that ended more than two decades ago and to Jo Ann's that endures. I set aside Rebecca's baby book and pick up a small head scarf in a plastic bag labeled "First gift from George," which he mentioned in a letter buying for her in NYC his first Christmas there. I pull it from the bag and wrap it around my neck.

I lift the tray and set it aside. Photographs, both prints and slides, are stacked in the cavity, some in shoe boxes, some in the envelopes and boxes they came in, some loose. Most of the containers are labeled: friends, family, house and yard, mountains. I groan. There are boxes and drawers and closets in this house filled with photographs and duplicates of photographs and photocopies of photographs, and now here are more. I pick up a sheet of wallet-size and two three-by-fives of my worst ever school picture—ninth grade. Three large manila envelopes labeled with my name and each of my sisters' names are filled with letters and postcards written home from college and years following, the entombed grains of our lives.

I leaf through photos of Mama and me in years I don't remember: holding the infant me in the rocking chair that is still in her bedroom and looking at eight-year-old me with delight in an alpine meadow—Mt. Rainier behind us. I hold the Rainier photo and let it take me back to picnics at Paradise: eating the tuna sandwiches, potato chips, and homemade chocolate chip cookies my mother had prepared and packed into the metal Coleman cooler—which is on a shelf above me—the grey jays and chipmunks grabbing food off our paper plates. I had a beautiful childhood, and my mother's love is at the root of it, hidden from view in the soil of today.

There are no letters in the trunk. I slump in disappointment.

I pull out the last box in the back corner—a square faded blue-green gift box tied up in white cotton string. A label on the lid says "Photos of and by Stellajoe before George."

I'm breathless as I lift it out and hold it unopened in my lap. I reload the trunk, push it back to the wall, and put the stuff back on top. It's past my bedtime, but I carry the box to my bedroom. I fold the scarf, putting it on my dresser next to a photograph of my father in his army uniform, and put on my pajamas. In bed, I untie the string and set aside the split-cornered lid, once held together by long gone cellophane tape, the residue discoloring the cardboard. Some of the packets have notes on the envelopes, but only a few photographs have identifying information on the back.

In the first envelope is image evidence of the rowboat with the little motor my mother owned with friends that my father mentions several times in his letters, inquiring if they still have it. I'm euphoric! My mother is holding the oars, like she's in charge. Who was this woman? In another, my young and vital girl-mother and her sister and a friend are walking through a meadow toward the camera, a river in the background, holding great armloads of daisies. A note on the back indicates that the land is the family farm of her friends—the sisters who owned the boat with her. The farm, my mother's handwriting indicates, is being flooded by the new Cherokee Dam. I hold the black-and-white photo in my hands, the image blurring through the tears that fill my eyes. I mourn this young woman I never knew, the years when her life was all ahead of her. I weep for the age-worn body and the depression that has robbed her of this unfettered joy.

I pull out a photograph of my mother with her sister at the 1939 New York World's Fair, standing straight and tall, stylish in pumps and tight-waisted full skirts, carrying patent leather handbags in white-gloved hands.

I open an envelope of pictures at Myrtle Beach, South Carolina. She has told me in past storytelling she drove there with a friend, borrowing her father's first ever car and breaking off the radio antennae. She was frightened to tell her father, she said, but he wasn't angry. There wasn't a radio in the car anyway.

She is wearing her Aunt Fannie's white terrycloth bathrobe as a beach robe, the one another photo shows her aunt wearing. In that photo, my mother is leaning against her aunt's shoulder on a sofa reading *Gone with the Wind*. The robe is unsashed in the beach photo, the front billowing open in the breeze, revealing her skirted swimming suit on her trim body. Wearing round sunglasses, her rag-curled long hair tossed from her face as she throws her head back, smiling broadly, she is beautiful and vital. My heart fills with love for this unknown woman.

I try to imagine when her life had beginnings and not endings. I wonder if she thinks about that. The photos help me let her out from behind the dim looking glass I have put her behind. I can see who she used to be, but I can't quite keep her there, the bent body and the complaining always in the forefront. I wonder if these years will fade when she is gone and if I will be able to free her from the prison of old age in my memory so I can carry the wholeness of her life in my heart.

I prop the daisy photograph against the lamp on my bedside table. Turning out the light, I sink beneath the covers to dream of the daisy meadows of my own long ago youth, brought closer because this house full of memories lives on.

∾

In the morning, I ask Mama about the photos I found. She confirms the note on the back of the daisy image.

"You were on the water, in a rowboat, as the lake was rising?" I ask, incredulous.

"I guess so," she says. "The next day we went back and drifted in the boat over the daisies swaying under the water covering what had been the rolling farm fields where we had walked the day before, rescuing what we could." I smile at that. My mother the daisy rescuer, like me before the lower part of the property gets its annual mowing.

"Tell me about the World's Fair with Doris," I press her.

"Doris wasn't there," she says.

"She's in the photo," I say.

"That's impossible," she insists. I want to show her the proof, but she can't see the images.

"There's one of you reading *Gone with the Wind*," I say, moving on and holding up the photo. I know it was a favorite book and remember when we went to see a re-release of the movie when I was nine, I was so terrified during the burning of Atlanta my father had to take me to the lobby.

She tells me she was eager to finish it before the movie came out in 1939. I have a hard time wrapping my head around the book and the movie being new. She's been on the earth for such a long time. But then I can't believe I've been alive long enough to know a time before a television in every living room and a microwave in every kitchen—or any kitchen.

I ask her about the photo of her in a swimming suit with a young man who isn't my father—she hadn't met him yet—his arm around her waist on the wet sand, the ocean behind them.

"Who is this?"

"Oh, I guess there were a couple of guys we met on the beach," she says.

"What was his name?" I prod.

"I don't remember. Maybe Bill something. I probably never knew his last name." It's hard to fathom that she had a life before my father, that she was someone who picked up guys, but in my hands is the evidence.

Here is her voice telling me she remembers more than she has thought about for a very long time. I know she has hundreds more stories, and I want to hear them all. But she can't think of them without the prompts I don't know to offer. I pick out more photos later, but she quickly tires of the game. I don't know if she really doesn't remember, or if remembering is painful.

45

June

Return

Mama was sure there was a better caregiver "out there" when the storm blew in six months ago, so she was happy when Michelle resigned, the non-firing firing. Five caregivers later, she may realize perfection doesn't exist.

"Michelle had good qualities," she says.

"She adored you," I say in agreement, "and she knew how you liked things done."

"She was clean in the kitchen," Mama says, getting at what's important. She doesn't say the good qualities made up for what she lacked: she wasn't a five-star cook, and when she did something that wasn't on The List, though it needed to be done, Mama felt robbed of control, and that irritated her. She doesn't say it because she has forgotten. She begins tearily to yearn to have Michelle back. "I didn't fire her," she repeats, as if trying to separate herself from blame for losing her.

When Mama learns what she had been smelling in her current caregiver's car since her first day of employment is that she has three dogs and four children who ride in the car, I hear her tell people, "I'm allergic." I'm not sure if she thinks she's allergic to the children or only the dogs, but she is sure that's what has caused the eye irritation she has struggled with since January, taking us to the eye doctor six times in six months before my WebMD diagnosis of a blocked tear duct is confirmed by the optometrist. That the caregiver and her car didn't come until March is lost on her. She has lost all sense of relative time.

Anticipating an imminent need for another caregiver to replace the current one, I have already contacted the Agency on Aging for resources, but on a whim I decide to call Michelle. It's unlikely she's available, and less likely she would want to come back, but why leave the stone unturned.

She *is* available, looking for a morning client in fact. But, she reminds me, the agency won't allow her to come back. "Hypothetically," I push, "if you could, would you want to? If you want to, do you think there's a way around the policy?" I tell her things will be different. I will be more involved and my mother will have to be okay with that. She will work for me, not for Mama, but that will be our little secret. She says she will think about it over the weekend and call her supervisor on Monday.

She calls me first thing Monday morning, soon after I arrive in Seattle for Elliot care. She wants to try, and her supervisor has reluctantly agreed to a two-week trial. I cheer wildly in my head, pumping my fist in the air.

ᘯ

Rebecca and I sit down with Mama when I return from Seattle and give her the news. She is overcome with emotion. We schedule time the next day when we are all rested to talk about what will be different to make the relationship successful.

The conversation goes better than I anticipated. "We are a team,"

I tell her, "you, me, Rebecca, Michelle, and Stan. We are working together to make you and me able to stay at home together. I will be checking in with Michelle and she with me on a regular basis. It's a condition of the rule waiver by the agency." She nods but says nothing. "Try to think of Michelle as a companion, a member of the team, rather than an employee," I suggest to deaf ears.

"If you want to sit on the deck and tell stories," Rebecca picks up, "let that be okay. We want you to have as much joy in your life as possible. You don't have to fill every moment with tasks." We know that will never happen. Paying someone to help you be happy is a squandering of money, in Mama's opinion. Maybe it's why she would never see a therapist for her chronic depression.

"But I'm spending your inheritance," she moans. "I've lived too long."

"It's not our inheritance until you're gone," I say. "It's your money to spend on your care. Besides, you have held onto and cared for this property for us. That's our inheritance. If we can keep you here, it makes us happy."

∽

Michelle starts the following week while I'm back in Seattle. "There was lots of hugging and crying," Rebecca reports.

When I see Michelle after my return, I ask her how it's going.

"Really well," Michelle says; "she's different. She's much kinder. And she isn't micromanaging. She goes to the living room and sits in her chair while I clean up the kitchen, rather than hovering to make sure I do it right. Everything is great. I know it might not last, but I'm in a better place too, and I think I'm back in it until the end. I love your mom."

I let out my breath.

year four

46

July

Anniversary

On the third anniversary of my drift down the driveway into my new life, I sit in the barn door with my coffee as the sun slides up through the trees across the meadow. I locate the red-breasted sapsucker on the utility pole drumming a loud accompaniment to the Cooing Dove Duo in the woods behind me. Two does and three spotted fawns shop for green apples in the orchard across the driveway, then split up. One jumps over the fence into my meadow, her baby close behind. The other family trots down the driveway, perhaps in hopes of a floral dessert at the house.

Coffee mug empty, I pick peas and chard from the garden, then return to the house, walking past the sweet-scented honeysuckle my mother has nurtured for many years, training it to grow on the fence and trying to keep the deer from eating it.

Mama is up and dressed when I return, and in the kitchen. Seventeen-month-old Elliot and his moms are still in bed after a late night in traffic getting to us. Elliot is being left in our care for three days while Emma and Wynne drive to Canada for the Women's World Cup soccer final and a much-needed break from parenting. He screams, red-faced, in my arms as they drive away, reaching his arms out after them.

When they are out of sight, I take him and his weeping heart to the garden.

"Look here, sweet boy," I say, and pick two sun-warmed strawberries for him. He takes a last shuttering gasp and eats them, pleasure spreading across his face. I open a pea pod and kneel in front of him, holding it out. He picks out the peas and pops them one at a time into his mouth.

"Mmmm," he says, pulling another from the vine.

That afternoon, Mama sits on the deck, something she rarely does, playing with Elliot in the water-play table I picked up at Goodwill. He grabs a duck and bends down, tilting his head to see her eyes under her visor. "Nana!" he shouts, and holds out the duck. She opens her hands and he gives it to her.

"What is this, Elliot?" she asks, her voice full of light.

"Duck!" he shouts, laughing as he snatches it back and plops it in the water.

The splash hits her in the face and she laughs back.

From my chair across the deck, I smile at their tacit understanding of each other. He is the antidote to this stifling life for both of us.

∾

A few days after Elliot goes back home, taking his light with him, I'm sitting in the chair in the corner of the living room when Mama, up from her nap, comes into the room. She doesn't sense my presence as she settles into her recliner with her hot water. Always cold, even in July, she puts the heating pad on her knees and covers her legs with an afghan. She has forgotten the visor that usually hides her face from view. I look at her in repose and can see how she has aged in the three years since I arrived. Her deeply wrinkled skin stretches across her facial bones, making her cheekbones more prominent. Her skin hangs loosely from her jowls. Her thin white hair, which I forgot to offer to put the curling iron to the last time she washed it, gives her a wild look. Her lips spread over her always large teeth that now seem too big for her mouth.

She reaches for the CD player I got her for Christmas and turns it on. I was skeptical that it would be of use to her, since she can't slow it down or back it up to understand a recorded book. But she can listen to music, though she rarely does, and she learned how to turn it on and adjust the volume. Fritz Kreisler—her favorite classical violinist, whom she listened to on the radio, waiting for her husband to return from the war—is on the player. She leans her head back and closes the eyes that have so betrayed her. She looks weary, perhaps of having to be here, living this greatly diminished existence. She is beautiful again as her face relaxes, giving up for a few moments the exhaustion of fighting with old age—and with me—to stay in control. I vow again to try to do what I can to give her that peace more often in our dealings with one another, knowing that if that means letting her be in control, it will continue to challenge me to the core.

In these three years, I've become more sure living here is the right thing to be doing, less sure it is the right thing to be doing; more understanding, more frustrated; more unsure that I can continue doing it, and more determined to hang on. But I'm tired, and as it becomes more clear that I must be vigilant about self-care, it becomes more difficult to do so. Twice this week, Mama became upset because she couldn't reach me, once forgetting how to use the phone, the next time forgetting to try. I was no farther away than the back garden, pulling weeds and breathing in momentary freedom.

She has become more accustomed to my presence as time passes, and is more quickly irritated with me. She's more irrational, more negative, more obsessive. She is more in need of ways to make her life more tenable, and more resistant to trying anything my sisters and I come up with to help her. In three years, the only thing she has let me completely take over is, finally, bill paying.

I try to keep it all together beneath her radar, allowing her to believe she is holding it together by herself, and I am—as my father used to joke of himself—just a necessary evil. I have to believe she knows deep down it is more than my presence in the basement that is keeping her at home, but she has never been one to throw praise out willy-nilly, even in my childhood, which is probably why I still crave being told I am appreciated and doing a good job. I have to depend on my sisters and friends for affirmation, and I still want it from my mother.

I've been here a thousand days, just about as long as John Kennedy was president, I realize, recalling the title of a book that used to be in the bookcase. I will serve longer than he did.

47

July

Magic Potion

"**G**rehhhhtchuuunnn." I'm not as startled as I used to be when the plaintive call comes over the monitor. It's six o'clock on the dot, a sure sign Mama has been waiting for a decent hour to summon me, and I don't need to break a leg to get to her. A bowel crisis, real or imagined, is an annual event. It's always on a weekend and often when there is only one daughter in town. Rebecca is on well-deserved R & R on the other side of the state.

I sigh and roll out of bed, picking up my glasses and phone and taking thirty seconds to scoop food into Smudge's bowl before I two-step it up the stairs. My gut sinks, knowing what's coming. I know she is hurting, I know it terrifies her, and I'm sad for her. How does she keep going? It's also hard to know what's real and what she is exaggerating.

"What's happening?" I ask her when I arrive at her bedside at 6:02.

"I don't want to, but I think I need to go to the emergency room."

"Well, let's try to avoid that. What's going on?"

"I haven't slept all night. I might have had too much exercise yesterday."

"Probably not," I say. Then, not waiting for her to tell me what hurts, I add, "In any case, I doubt it would give you abdominal pain."

"Or maybe too much Miralax."

"Nope," I say.

"Maybe it's a parasite. Maybe I ate a peach with a worm in it."

She farts, and I suggest maybe it's gas. She says nothing. She's not interested in any theory that won't get her to the ER, in spite of what she says. She continues to moan, make demands, and refuse every suggestion to make her more comfortable. She carries on an argumentative conversation with herself:

"I need to go to the ER, but only to the one in Olympia."

"I don't think I can sit up in the car to get there."

"The ambulance won't take me there unless I go to Centralia first."

"I'm not going to Centralia."

"The Centralia hospital will want to take X-rays. I don't like X-rays."

She must confuse even herself. I tell her any ER will take X-rays for a presenting problem of stomach distress and with her history. I call the on-call care provider at her doctor's office and, in a stroke of luck, it's Mama's doctor. She doesn't think it sounds like an obstruction and suggests urgent care—an option we haven't tried before.

"I can't go to urgent care," Mama says; "they don't take X-rays."

Her confusion concerns me more than her discomfort. I tell her we're going to try it, cutting off negotiations.

∽

I try to keep her comfortable until they open as I note a lack of the usual blockage symptoms. Right off she tells the X-ray technician she doesn't like X-rays and he can only do one, a last gasp effort to run the show, forgetting her assertion that they don't do X-rays. He ignores her, of course, and takes what he needs. There is no visible blockage. The tentative diagnosis is dehydration, maybe gas. The doctor suggests Gatorade.

We stop at the grocery store on the way home. She takes two sips of Gatorade and says she feels much better. An orange magic potion.

We remain on stormy seas for the next week. Mama doesn't dress, spends most of the time lying down, eats only because I insist, and doesn't poop. She drinks quarts of Gatorade.

She tells me a dream.

"There was a nuclear disaster, or something, and the air was full of smoke. We were walking to the ocean, hoping there would be breathable air there. Thousands of people. There was a grandstand where people were sitting, to rest maybe. Someone way at the top dropped a pendant with an Indian design on it. It fell at my feet. I picked it up and held it up so she could see that I had it. She found me later, and stayed with me; sometimes carrying me on her back. I thought it was my mother, and I looked into many rooms for her, then saw her in the distance at the top of a hill with her walker. I waved to her, but she didn't see me."

I have read that paying attention to the dreams of the elderly gives important clues about what is coming and what goes on, unspoken, inside of them. They often sense what is coming, and—if they try to tell us—we are apt to be dismissive. She saw her mother, but her mother didn't seem to see her. It's not yet time for her to go—the antithesis of being beckoned. It was dark, smoky, hard to breath—the antithesis of the bright light we hear spoken of in near-death stories. Maybe she's getting ready, but she's not leaving yet.

On Thursday, I have a flash of realization: her mother died

thirty-two days after her ninety-ninth birthday. Sunday, the day of the crisis, was thirty-one days after Mama's ninety-ninth birthday. She has finally outlived her mother. I wonder if there is subconscious awareness.

∾

Fixing her breakfast is one of the last things Mama can do independently. She needs help, but she won't ask for it nor accept my offers. This morning the water for her hot cereal cools while she heats her milk. While she reheats the water and mixes up the cereal, the milk gets too cool. While she heats more milk, the cereal gets cold. When she gets it to the table and realizes she has "failed," she collapses in tears of frustration. I offer to make it again for her, but she says she will do it herself.

She tells me another dream. "I was on the ocean in a boat, and there was a wild storm all around me, and I was trying to get three small children to a safer place." There is no one left she needs to protect, she's becoming the cared for. She's desperately trying to hang on to the independence that keeps her safe, and she's failing. My heart hurts for her.

∾

Sunday morning she has a bowel movement. In celebration, she dresses and goes out to walk on the deck. I know she's back to herself when she asks me if she has ever told me the best placement in the dishwasher for the Pyrex custard dishes. "You have been telling me since 1962," I assure her.

48

July

Hospice

Following two early morning weekend crises in six weeks, I ask Mama's primary care doctor for a hospice referral. I know hospice is for people with a terminal diagnosis, and I don't understand how being ninety-nine isn't terminal. I need a nurse who will come to the house every week to listen to Mama's often irrational health fears, to assure her that she isn't having a heart attack, to determine if her abdominal pain is a blockage or gas. I don't want to take her to the doctor or the ER every time she panics. She doesn't want medical intervention for anything that ails her, but she doesn't trust my knowledge and intuition to tell her she's okay, and I don't always trust it either. I want to keep her home, but I need help.

When I lay out my case, the doctor says she is a perfect candidate. But for Medicare to pay, there must be a diagnosis with a 51 percent chance that the client *could* die from within six months. Merely being on the edge of a century old, which inherently puts one at risk of a life-changing event at any moment, is not of interest to Medicare. The doctor puts in a referral based on congestive heart failure, which her cardiologist now says she doesn't have. I learn not to confound the referral process with the facts. At ninety-nine, I suppose even

Medicare will understand there is a 51 percent chance of her heart stopping.

Not being able to perform basic self-care could help, and I learn not to tell the certifying hospice doctor she can dress herself, because someone has to help her find her clothes; not to say she can feed herself, because someone has to tell her what's on her plate; not to say she can bathe herself, because someone is always standing by. Nuanced truth-telling.

She gets in. I feel like we've won the lottery. I am unaware of the "evidence of decline" requirement to *keep* her in.

⌒

A few days after our acceptance, we meet Laurel, the nurse on our hospice team. She is a cheerful, pleasant-looking woman in her fifties with a long blond ponytail, wearing dark blue scrubs, not printed with kittens, thank goodness. She speaks directly to Mama and holds her hand as she checks in with her, then takes her vitals and listens to her bowel tones. They chat about Mama's health and history and Laurel tells her about her life on a horse farm. Laurel skillfully includes me in the conversation, while never excluding Mama.

When Mama tells her about the lorazepam in the hospital that robbed her of her vision, rather than telling Mama that's unlikely, she calls Mama's glaucoma doctor and asks if it's possible. *Damn. She knows her stuff.*

She tells us she will come once a week for now, and she can come more often if needed. I don't even try to stop my tears of gratitude. Mama will have a place regularly to share her ongoing fears with someone with letters after their name. When the social worker, the chaplain, and the bath aide come in the next days, I feel a new energy. I'm doing this. I'm taking care of my mother and, albeit with the added task of scheduling the team around Mama's energy and their availability, and trying to avoid more than one of them a day, I'm taking care of myself too.

49

September

Grey

Stop the correspondence I'm coming home will leave Ansbach April 2 Love=George

After sixteen months intimately spent with my father through his letters, I return the final telegram to its protective sleeve and close the three-inch binder, ready to be added to the other five in the bookcase.

His spirit lives in this home he loved—in his workshop, the barn, the trees—but in the letters he was alive again. As my ancient mother slept, and the darkness out the windows turned to light each morning, I immersed myself in his words, his familiar handwriting, his humor, his intelligence. Now the letters are finished, and I am grieving him all over again.

I saw the mother I know in the letters. The maddening personality traits didn't just materialize in old age. But I also saw a side of her I never knew, or don't remember. I wonder if that adventurous person with a zest for life and love is still buried deep inside. With the completion of the letters, I will grieve the loss of her vibrance.

Jo Ann comes for a visit so I can get away with my tent. I knew it was going to rain, but I couldn't bear not to go. I changed my reservation from the remote Takhlakh Lake to Lake Quinault in the Olympic Peninsula's temperate rain forest. It isn't quite glamping, but the amenities of flush toilets and potable water put it in a class beyond most of my camping experiences of past years. The campground is a half mile walk from the historic lodge with a writing desk by the fire crackling in the enormous stone fireplace. I drink tea and write and watch the rainclouds drape over the lake through the tall windows.

Mama and I had a pair of mini-vacations here when I came home for visits in years past. I have lunch one day at the table we always sat at in the dining room named for FDR—the third-term president Mama marked her first ballot for—in honor of his visit in 1937, prior to signing the Olympic National Park into being. I sit facing the lake and the hummingbird feeders that hang from the eaves, across from her chair with her back to the light, and order the salmon burger that Mama said wasn't dinner. I am never far from her past and our history together.

～

I return home to a sunny week with autumn in the air. I'm ready to put the garden to bed and hunker inside and watch the rain. Mama doesn't like fall because it comes before winter, and she hates winter. Living in the Pacific Northwest makes half the year—a season called Grey—challenging for those with seasonal depression. While I was gone, Laurel—who's been with us for several weeks now and has rapport with Mama—talked to Mama about depression while Jo Ann eavesdropped. Laurel posed it as anxiety, somehow knowing the word "depression" is a conversation-stopper for Mama. Stunningly she agreed to try an antianxiety medication.

This week, Laurel tells us she researched some medications, formulated for the elderly. Mama prevaricates. "It's not anything in me that is a problem," she says. "It's that my daughters don't understand my limitations, and they get angry and make me feel bad about myself." It's the external locus of control she has mastered over her decades, always something "out there" to blame. I'm sure "daughters" plural is code for "daughter" singular, and I'm ashamed to hear I make her feel bad about herself. I once again renew my intention to express more compassion, and know I will fail again.

Laurel talks to her about the value of expressing anger over stuffing it down, following up on a similar conversation with the hospice social worker, whom Mama clearly thought was full of crap. "Are you saying," Mama says, "I should respond to anger with anger?"

"Yes!" Laurel says. "It's not healthy to push it down."

It's enlightenment she has no use for. She's a lifetime stuffer, and she's not going to change now. My task is to accept her as she is. I didn't cause it, and I can't fix it. I should write the reminder in lipstick on my bathroom mirror.

I walk Laurel to the door, where she stops and, turning to me says, "I've got some bad news."

She's leaving, I think. *Shit.*

"Unless something happens in the next month, I won't be able to keep her in hospice. She's too healthy."

I stop breathing. Laurel had explained Medicare's "declining" requirement, but it's a fact I've conveniently kept from lodging in my brain.

"I'm sorry. Being a family caregiver is hard and it's always good to have an outsider involved, but Medicare doesn't care about that. If your mama will agree to the antidepressant, that could keep her in while we get it regulated."

But Mama doesn't like drugs. She won't take the antidepressant, in spite of agreeing to it. I close my eyes and dream of my tent and the cozy lodge.

⤳

"It is 1:03 a.m."

"It is 1:03."

"It is 1:03 a.m."

Shit! With a sigh, I roll over, knocking the cat off my legs as I lean over to turn on the video of the monitor I got to replace the original cheap buzzing one. Mama appears to be asleep. Her talking clock stops its robotic announcement. I pull the covers back up and Smudge settles back down.

"It is 1:05 a.m."

"It is 1:05."

Smudge jumps off the bed and goes to check her food bowl.

"It is 1:10 a.m."

"It is 1:10."

"It is 1:10 a.m."

Dammit! I drag myself out of bed and trudge upstairs. Mama's sleeping with her hand on the clock's large button, or maybe she isn't asleep. I pull it out from under her fingers and move it out of reach. She'll be unhappy when she can't find it, but not pushing the button when it's dark out was a condition of having the clock in bed with her at night. I return to bed. Neither Smudge nor I go back to sleep.

I look out the window into the darkness. The valley is filled with fog, blocking light from the trailer park below. The stars are bright. I spot Orion at the edge of the fir tree. Through the open window, I hear geese calling and answering in the blankness, trying not to get lost, perhaps. A coyote howls and starts a ruckus.

I keep my eyes on Orion's belt, thinking about my life, lost but for these touchstones of beauty and comfort that get me through. The talking clock is Mama's touchstone. One by one, the three stars blink out as the fog dissipates and the lights from the ground fade them. I drift off to sleep.

❧

I head to Seattle a few hours later for a play day with Elliot. I haven't spent a day with him since school ended for Wynne in mid-June, and my year of Mondays and Tuesdays with him concluded. She's back at school now, and he's playing hooky from day care to play with me. I'm tired from the interrupted night, but the prospect of seeing him—and an extra caffeine shot in my road latte—sparks my energy for the drive.

When I pull up to the curb opposite their house, he and Emma meet me at the end of the driveway. Elliot puffs out his chest, proudly showing me the T-shirt he's wearing emblazoned with the words, "Big Brother." It takes me a minute. Then I look at Emma, wide-eyed.

"You're pregnant?" I exclaim.

"Due in May," she says, touching her stomach.

I want to do cartwheels, but I settle for swinging Elliot into my arms and hugging Emma—and my new grandchild—tight. Elliot and I have a beautiful day. I swear he said "Gigi" once. His sweet love lightens me, and the promise of a baby makes all right in my universe.

50

September

Teetering on the Edge

The morning after my return from Seattle, Rebecca calls to ask if I can work at her shop for her on Monday. She'll be out of town and also can't take her weekly turn cooking Mama's dinner. I won't get my Monday adventure day, but I say of course—she deserves a vacation—and hang up. I run upstairs without breakfast to greet Mama shortly before Laurel is due, and she tells me Laurel can't come today, but will come tomorrow—when I have yoga. Apparently I missed her call to me, so she called Mama, who told her that was fine.

"You have a manicure appointment on the calendar for that time," I tell her. "Do you want to cancel it?"

"I don't want to cancel it, because I need a haircut too."

"Did you tell them that? You can't make an appointment for one thing and expect them to have time for something else too." It's not the first time I've told her that when she's been put out not to get what she didn't ask for.

"No," she says. "Michelle can call and ask when she gets here. Maybe Laurel can come on Thursday. Do I have anything on Thursday?"

"Thursday is her day off, and I made an appointment for your flu shot."

"Friday, then. Do I have anything else on Friday?"

"We're going to Olympia to the ENT in the afternoon." The appointment was made to replace the hearing aid remote that was lost and now is found, but she wants to keep the appointment because maybe this time there will be a magic fix for her profound hearing loss. "And you wanted to reschedule the reader." She canceled the hospice volunteer because the reader from the church was coming. She canceled him because the hospice reader was coming. She didn't ask for scheduling help.

"And when is my ENT appointment?"

"Friday."

"And when is my flu shot?"

"Thursday."

"That's three things on Thursday. That's too much." It's really four, the bath aide is coming early on Thursday too, but I don't bring that up. "But when is the ENT? I thought that was Thursday."

"That's on Friday."

"Is that all that's on Friday?"

"Yes."

"When is the nurse coming?

"Wednesday, if we cancel your manicure," I say, resigning myself to missing yoga.

"And what else is Wednesday?"

"You said you wanted the reader to come in the afternoon."

"Isn't the ENT that afternoon?"

"No, it's on Friday. Can we cancel the manicure on Wednesday so the nurse can come?"

"I don't want to change the manicure if I can get a haircut at the same time. If I can't, you can cancel the manicure."

Michelle arrives and deals with the salon. I deal with the hospice appointments while trying not to tear my hair out.

"You can get a haircut Friday morning," I tell Mama. "Is that okay? And keep Laurel on Wednesday?"

"What else is on Friday?"

"The ENT in the afternoon."

"I thought that was on Thursday." I bend forward and put my head in my hands. I'm either the best daughter on the planet for letting her be involved, or the worst, for not freeing her from herself.

I go back downstairs at ten fifteen for my much-delayed breakfast and remember I'm out of granola. I made it through the crazy-making conversation and accepted that next week is in shatters, and it's granola that sends me over the edge. A train rumbles through town in the distance and I howl on pitch with its whistle.

∿

Usually sleep will clear my head and heart, but I wake in the wee hours in tears. If I could figure out another option—any option—for my life, I would be plotting a new plan at this very moment. But I can't think of one. I feel stuck. My stomach stays in a knot from trying not to scream at Mama. From not having a life. From not having friends. From Mama believing I'm a freeloader she's taking care of so I'm not living under a bridge in a sleeping bag. What would happen to her, I wonder, if I stopped "freeloading"? Does she ever think of that?

∿

When I go upstairs the next morning—late again, this time because I didn't want to get out of bed—Mama has had trouble with her breakfast and berates me for not being there to help her, which she has never wanted me to do. "You don't do much in exchange for all you get by living here that you don't have to pay for," she says.

"Oh, I pay for it," I say.

Next week I'm getting a third crown since I've been here because I clench my teeth at night and crack the old fillings. It better be jewel studded.

51

November

New Terrain

I am in heaven, ensconced for a week in a tiny cottage at Hedgebrook, the iconic women's writing retreat center on Whidbey Island. We have two-and-a-half hours of writing instruction with a master teacher most days, and hours alone to read, write, and sleep. There is a tiny wood stove, a large desk, and a sleeping loft. The efficiency kitchen holds one set of flatware, one small plate and one large one, one mug, one water glass, one wine glass. I am just one here, with no one to care for other than myself.

Sumptuous dinners are prepared by the chef for the seven writers and our instructor, and I return to my Fir Cottage in the circle of light from my flashlight, seeing only what is two steps ahead. I carry a basket of what I need for breakfast and lunch the next day: an egg, a tablespoon of olive oil, ground coffee for the French press, a quarter cup of milk, two slices of Dave's Killer Bread—one for breakfast toast, one to go with delicious homemade soup for lunch—two pats of butter. When I finish my two meals, the refrigerator will be empty. This is how I want to live. With just enough to eat and just enough space.

I'm disappointed that my cottage has sporadic phone reception.

Rebecca texts that things aren't going well at home in my absence, that Mama is confused and anxious. I turn off my phone.

After a stormy day on Tuesday, the power is out for nearly twenty-four hours. The emergency light in my cottage goes out too, and the batteries in the flashlight die. I am alone in the dark. I get by on my inner compass, like I will get through this dark night with my mother. An owl in the woods speaks before dawn: "All will be well," she calls; "all will be well."

Waking to the patter of rain on the roof a few feet above my head in the loft each morning, I could stay in bed as long as I want—no cat walking on me, no clomping footfalls over my head— but I'm up at five thirty as always. I build a fire and make tea, then wrap in the afghan and sit on the window bench to wait for the fire to warm the cottage, not turning on the electric space heater. As I watch the day come, I read entries in the journals of those who stayed in Fir Cottage before me, including Gloria Steinem, a member of the board.

I walk on the path through the trees to the bath house. I fill the long, deep tub and in candlelight sink slowly under the water. I'm drowning. Does my mother feel like she's drowning? What is it like not to know when you go to bed at night if you will surface again? I wonder if I find compassion difficult because, with her decline in my face all the time, I fear my own march toward that slippery slope.

I want to stay in this cottage forever. I want just to stare out into the winter forest, not work on my writing project about life with my mother. Writing and sharing this life and hearing back from readers on similar journeys keeps me sane, but I wish I could leave it behind for this week. I've spent money—in my fantasies, saved for a trip to Italy—to come here; I need to make the most of the time. But what would be most?

Leave your expectations behind, I read in a ten-year-old journal entry. *We have enough put upon us in our regular lives. The time here is not for that. Relax. Don't worry so much. Whatever work you do here is the work you were supposed to do.* I hold onto the words on my drive home to my real life, hoping my work there is enough too.

∽

The week after my return, Mama is not herself. We are in a new land of confusion, agitation, fabrication, paranoia, and accusation. I'm grateful Jo Ann is still here, having come across the country again so I could be away.

Rebecca comes for breakfast on Jo Ann's last day. Laurel comes as scheduled, having astoundingly persuaded Mama to start an anti-depressant a couple of weeks ago, keeping us in hospice. Stan the Handy Man shows up to work, unscheduled. Mama wants to know where Michelle is. Jo Ann reminds her she told her not to come today. Mama denies it and claims to have called a "meeting of the team" for this morning. We are all mystified, but rather than argue I call Michelle and apologetically ask if she can come up the hill for an hour. We wait, gathered around the dining table, until Michelle arrives, Mama refusing to say a word until she gets here.

Mama takes control. She accusatorially recounts conversations and events of previous days in great detail: I said . . . she said . . . I did . . . this happened . . . they forgot.

"Don't correct her," Laurel whispers to us. "Just let her go."

Michelle is fighting tears. "That didn't happen," she murmurs.

"It's okay, honey," Laurel says quietly.

"We know it didn't happen," I say.

Mama goes around the table asking each of us a question in turn. "Did you do this . . . say this. . . ?" We each say yes without meaning yes. Stan says, "Yes, ma'am." Rebecca won't play and says what we all want to say: "That's not quite how I remember it," giving her version.

"I'm in charge!" Mama shouts. "You all work for me!"

Laurel puts her hand on Mama's and gently tells her we all love her, we all want her to be happy. "But right now you are being really mean to us, Stella. You are saying things that aren't true. How can we help you now?"

"I need Michelle to make me some lunch," Mama says. Michelle's eyes widen as she shakes her head.

"You gave Michelle the day off, Stella," Laurel says. "She made other plans."

"I'll make your lunch," Jo Ann jumps in. Mama slumps, spent and defeated.

At the door, Laurel affirms what David has told me: the long explanations of how Mama believes something went down is her attempt to tell herself she remembers details, though fabricated. We all think she's heading into her final decline. I'm terrified. Jo Ann leaves tomorrow, and I will be on my own. *For better for worse. In sickness and health. Till death do us part.*

I don't know how to respond when Mama tells me I did or said something I did not do or say. Or that she told me to do something she did not tell me to do, and so I hadn't done it, and now she is upset with me. It happens frequently over the next days.

On his "Age of Disruption Tour," Dr. Bill Thomas, gerontology expert and performer, says, "We have to meet them in the present, which requires a rewiring of sorts on our part. Our expectations must change." Mama's present is a hard place to be. I know I can't argue with dementia. Things stay calm when I say, "Okay," "You're right," or "I understand," when it doesn't feel okay, she's not right, and I do not understand. When I fight with my sword of rationality, the disagreement escalates until she shuts down. Implying that she is crazy robs her of dignity and serves no purpose. I am the worst daughter on the planet.

"It's better to be kind than right, and you will lose all points of fact anyway," is number five on my parental caregiver friend Elizabeth's "Top Ten Tips for Dealing with Dementia." Number ten is "drink more wine." I skip to the end.

⁓

Mama is aware something has changed. She remains tired and unsteady. I'm hanging onto hope her tumble down the rabbit hole is due to the stressors of the month—changing heating systems (getting rid of the fossil fuel furnace is one of my accomplishments), Michelle's vacation, my vacation, having Jo Ann here, all of which have disrupted routine—and that she will get back to herself. Laurel says it could be that.

Laurel is coming this morning, and I go upstairs early to make sure Mama gets her breakfast in time. She's sitting at the kitchen table with her hot water. I sit down in the other chair.

"Did you sleep well?" I ask.

"No," she says with a sigh. "And my vision is more blurry than ever. I don't think I can see to get my breakfast."

"I'll fix it for you," I tell her.

Laurel arrives while she's finishing her Cream of Wheat.

"How are you, Stella?" she asks brightly.

"I can't see and I'm tired all the time. It's the antidepressant. I'm not going to take it anymore!" she says emphatically, as Laurel pulls her blood pressure cuff from her bag.

"Could it possibly be the antidepressant?" I ask Laurel quietly.

"It's unlikely," she says. "It's very mild and she's taking a tiny dose. But if that's what she thinks it is, there is no point in continuing it."

Before she leaves, she tells me how to wean her off of it gradually, as all of us know that is how you have to stop using antidepressants. All of us except Mama.

༄

The next morning, I cut her half-pill dose in half again.

"I'm not going to take it," she says.

"It's important to taper off of them," I explain. "Otherwise you could have more severe side effects."

"Okay," she snarls, as she takes it from me and puts it in her mouth. It dawns on me that perhaps she has already abruptly stopped taking it and that is the cause of her symptoms rather than the drug itself.

She spits it out into her cloth napkin, trying to make me think she is spitting out food she can't eat. It's not how she has ever removed food from her mouth before, but I don't accuse her. I wonder if she's remembering my grandmother telling her she deceived her husband into thinking she was taking the herbal remedies he forced on her to end any potential pregnancy. I'm heartbroken to think she believes something is being forced on her against her will.

With each increasingly smaller dose and with decreasing frequency, I gently remind her why it's important to follow the instructions. She never responds, and continues to spit the pill into her napkin.

Her behavior is increasingly erratic over the next week.

"She's not taking it," I report to Laurel.

"Let it go," she says. "She's going to do what she wants to do. You all will suffer for it, but she will even out."

When she is back to normal, she confesses she didn't take the pills. "I know," I say. There is no point in telling her she made it harder on herself.

Friends, trying to be helpful, tell me their parent had good results with this or that drug, including the storied lorazepam. I know doctors experiment with antidepressants until they find what works and at what dose, and I know Mama will never agree to try another one. Depression and disappointment are what she knows. She's comfortable with it. I don't know if I can stop being at war with it, but it's her battle, not mine. *You didn't cause it, you can't fix it,* I repeat to myself.

⌒⌣

When Michelle arrives the next day, I put on a jacket and go out in the weak winter sun to my father's workshop over the carport. Turning on my electric fireplace in the room at the back, I shed my jacket and curl up with the afghan in my red leather chair with a cup of tea and let my mind wander.

A friend who lives with her mother's Alzheimer's says it's like living with a ghost. She says she will be relieved when her mother dies, and I love her for that honesty. She asks if I will be relieved when my mother dies. The first thing that zips through me is, "God, yes," but then I realize there is a lot more to it than that. When I moved back here, I thought maybe we could stop being the parent and the child and be friends. I realize now we will never have that relationship. We are too different. Or too the same.

I read somewhere that in the months before the death of a loved one, we need to let go of all those things we wish we had or thought we needed in our relationship with them, but didn't get. It's too late. "Turn the tables and *give* what you didn't get but still need," the article suggested. That gives me pause. Do I fight against giving unconditional love and acceptance to my mother because she withholds them from me? I'm probably not the daughter she wishes she had, either.

I want her to stop being my mother, and let me be an adult, but I'm acting like a child.

At once I know, I *will* grieve when she's gone. I will grieve the foreverness of giving up on my longing to have a champion, a mother who could express head-over-heels pride in me, a mother I wanted to share everything with, a mother I knew as a best friend. When she's gone, any hope of transformation goes too.

For now, though, it's time for me to shed the child that lurks in me and to validate myself. I will keep striving to accept my mother as the mother I got and release her from my fantasy. Maybe it's only when she's gone that I will be able forgive her for not being that mother—and myself for not being that daughter. In life we do battle against the ghosts of what will never be, but death will come, bringing with it the last word.

52

February

Leaving Before the Rains Come

Mama's name is still on the waiting list at the assisted living residence. The director has called a couple times since I moved home, and each time Mama said no, she didn't want the room. When Ellen calls me today, I think the room has become available again. But she and I talked informally a few months ago and determined Mama needs more care now than they provide. It isn't why she's calling. She's going through the waiting list, and wonders if my mother should be removed and her hundred-dollar deposit refunded. It's a milestone decision. She confirms her opinion that Mama would not thrive there now and, without consulting anyone, including Mama, I tell her to remove her from the list her name has occupied for over a decade.

I wonder if being surrounded by peers, people who are in the same boat, appealed to Mama. If she had gone sooner, would she have learned to enjoy new things and let go of trying to do what she no longer can, or would she have given up and died? Aging at home is what we hope for, for ourselves and our parents. But is it always best? Because they are at home doesn't mean they are thriving. There is no ideal, so we pick an option and hang on for the ride until we need to change boats.

When I tell Mama her sister-in-law who lives in the Arizona desert—the one she lived with in Michigan when their husbands were overseas in WWII—who has broken many bones over the years and is sinking into dementia, has moved to assisted living, she weeps. "I'm so lucky!" she sobs as I hold her. I take it as affirmation that she doesn't regret the decision we made to keep her at home. But for how long? It's magical thinking that she is not going to decline and can stay at home indefinitely. We still haven't formed a plan for the future. We're still holding our breath against a catastrophic event, risking being caught completely unprepared.

∾

This property is the keeper of both natural history and my history. While Mama struggles to maintain the illusion of control, I work harder than I want to keep the four acres from returning to wilderness. I beat back the salal and blackberry vines to reach the big leaf maple that once held the tree house my father built for his grandchildren, its trunk holding ash from the 1980 eruption of Mt. St. Helens deep in its layers. There are bits of the old wooden fence that surrounded the meadow when I was a child, falling down in what is now woods but wasn't then. Even the "new" fence my father and Nicholas were building when my father went to the hospital and never came home has become worn and lichen covered—as everything is in the Pacific Northwest. The new vegetable garden will soon be replanted for its third season, and the hostas I planted in the side yard where Mama warned nothing would grow have pushed their way through the moss for their rebirth.

I spend today in the sunshine, thinning the bud-filled

flowering quince. The juncos that rest in community in its thick maze of branches return to their solitary work searching for bugs and seeds in the grass. It's my third pass at this long-abandoned bush. I snip off shoots, saving the longest ones to weave into my garden fence to keep the deer out. My mother has done a stunning job of taking care of the house and flower beds, but her philosophy of the property beyond the parameters of the yard has been that she doesn't want it to look like a park. Maybe that was code for "I can't do it all, something has to go."

As I prune the quince, I wonder how long I will want to stay on this land. My mother has had an isolated life here since my father died; is that what I want? Should I get out of here when my mother is gone and get established in a town house in an urban neighborhood instead of pruning a bush no one will see except me and the juncos? Like wondering when to move Mama, I have no answer.

But something shifts in me as I work. A flicker begins *tap-tap-tapping* in the ancient big leaf maple next to the house; the returning geese honk down the rain-flooded valley under blue skies; I can almost smell the apples that will form on the trees down the slope. This is who I am. I am not an apartment-in-town person, content to replace last season's pansies with summer's impatiens in a planter box by the front stoop or to tend to well-behaved gardens, and neither was my mother.

This morning the sun split the dark sky behind the mountain and striped it pink, and nothing else mattered but my curiosity about what would happen next. And then it's gone, and the shades of grey take over, and there is nothing left to show for it except the pictures I took, the tears I wept at its beauty, the fullness of my heart.

I'm sure this is why my mother stayed. She couldn't bear to leave the sunrise and the woodpeckers behind. Just as she must often have doubted her decision, there will be days I will think this was the dumbest one I ever made, when the winter wind storms across the hillside, and I'm afraid of falling trees; when my back aches from the spring work that keeps me from my writing. And there are other days the sunrise and the smell of the earth after rain will leave me without words. When it's time to move on, I will, but for now I'm glad I said yes to this adventure. And I'm glad Mama is still here too.

53

March

Flunking Hospice

"I forgot to tell him about the melanomas," Mama says after the hospice social worker leaves.

"He's not medical staff," I tell her for the umpteenth time.

"I thought he was a doctor," she says.

"No, social worker," I say. I should have left it at that. "And you don't have any melanomas."

"Who told you that!" she demands.

"The dermatologist."

"Well, you must have made that up. They biopsied something."

"That's right," I say, ignoring her implication that I am the one with dementia. "And three months later we went back to have it checked, and the sample he took for biopsy turned out to be all there was. He said it was gone."

"But there are several more," she insists.

"They are all precancerous," I say, reminding her that he froze them.

"They don't know that; they didn't send any others in for testing."

"That's because they weren't suspicious," I say, trying and failing to keep frustration out of my voice. She shuts down.

It's a futile conversation, and we've had it before, but she continues to tell the hospice staff she has several "cancerous melanomas." She tells my aunt on the phone, talking slowly, her volume increasing with each repetition, trying to make her ninety-three-year-old sister understand an imagined ailment while her sister simultaneously shouts her own misfortunes that I can hear across the room. It's sadly hilarious.

༺

Rebecca comes up for dinner this evening. While we eat, Mama tells us in stunning detail about the recorded book she's listening to on the diets of the world's longest-lived people.

"What interests you in the topic?" I ask.

"I'm wondering what I should be eating," she says. Rebecca and I exchange a wide-eyed look, smothering laughter.

"Are you going to start drinking red wine?" Rebecca asks, a finding Mama didn't mention.

"Are you going for oldest person in the world?" I ask.

"I don't want to live any longer!" she assures me, ignoring Rebecca's comment.

I look sidewise at Rebecca, who returns my glance. I'm imagining the entry in Guinness.

Since Mama was admitted into hospice care, she is eating better and has become stronger. Laurel is coming tomorrow and we are up for recertification again after gaining some time with the failed antidepressant trial. I'm sure she will flunk out.

༺

My chest is tight with anxiety as Laurel sits down at the table across the corner from Mama. Rebecca has joined us and sits next to me.

"Well," she says after she takes Mama's vitals—which are perfect, as always—"I have bad news."

Here it comes. I close my eyes. I want to shut my ears.

"I just can't keep you in hospice any longer, Stella," she says.

Mama looks as stricken as I feel. I hear Rebecca's sharp intake of breath.

The discharge papers read: "1. No symptoms of recurrent congestive heart failure. 2. No debilitating chest pain. 3. Class II (mild) of the NY Heart Association Classification of Heart Failure. 4. No supportive criteria: no temporary loss of consciousness due to a drop in blood pressure, no anorexia, no oxygen dependence, no general bedbound status."

In other words, failure to decline.

"It's a good thing!" Laurel says, patting Mama's bony hand. "You are doing so well!"

"Spin it any way you want, but it's not a good thing," I say, trying to keep the bitterness out of my voice. It's not Laurel's fault.

"It's not uncommon for patients to improve while under hospice care," she says. "It's the best insurance around, but Medicare hasn't figured that out."

"There needs to be a program for people who live too long," Rebecca says.

"There needs to be program for children of people who live too long," I say under my breath.

I would be glad if Mama accepted her well-being, but she desperately wants something to be wrong and someone to act sympathetic, which is not me. I need someone to call when she says she needs to go to the ER. I need someone who will listen to her talk as often as she wants to about the decades old hematoma inside her left elbow; someone who will hypothesize, again, that the pain in her earlobe is probably from the pressure of sleeping on it, not from whatever she imagines it is; someone who will tell her that her ankles aren't swollen, her lungs are strong, her oxygen levels are perfect, contrary to what she thinks, and that she needs to keep taking her Miralax. Someone other than me, because I have no credibility. If the ailments she makes up could keep her in, we would be golden.

I especially don't want her to lose the bath aide, the highlight of her week. The thought of that loss sends me spiraling into panic.

I'm grateful to the hospice team for getting us through winter—Mama's blue season—keeping us in the program through the two previous six-week re-certifications. Laurel assures us we can get back in anytime her doctor refers her, and we will be assigned the same team. Today I can't Pollyanna the blow away. I feel abandoned. I burst into tears. I'm on my own again.

I'm drinking Mama's red wine.

54

April

Obsession

Mama hangs onto regret like barnacle to rock. Her ongoing obsession is that she didn't appreciate her mother's hard life and sacrifice and didn't respect her in her old age. That her mother was a difficult old woman is not what she remembers. That she did the best she could is not enough, won't ever be enough. She put her on a pedestal after she died in 1988, and there she will stay. Maybe that's what all daughters do to their mothers, realizing their virtue only after they are gone.

"Someday you will understand what it's like to be old, Gretchen," she tells me this morning. "I don't want you to live the rest of your life wishing you had understood me better, like I have wished about my mother."

"I wish you could let it go," I say to deaf ears. What I am determined to remember, in spite of any regrets, is that I did the best I could, and if I had it to do over, my best is still all I could have done. I know it's not always enough.

"You don't know what it's like to be blind," she says. "You don't know what it's like to have to be careful of what you eat."

"No, I don't know what it's like," I say. "Tell me."

"I can't see to cook my egg."

"Yes, but how does it feel? Are you afraid? Do you want to collapse in tears? Do you wish you could die? Do you long for the past? Is your young woman self still inside you?" I want to plumb the depths of her feelings, open her up and dive into the turbid pool. But her emotions are padlocked, and she has thrown away the key. Even she can't unlock them.

"I just want my egg cooked soft," she says.

∾

My mother grew up poor in East Tennessee. She was the second of four children born to her mother, and the eighth to her previously widowed father who didn't want more children and used cruel means in foiled attempts to end possible pregnancies in his determined, twenty-years-younger wife.

They moved fourteen times in her childhood—to and from houses without electricity or plumbing—to avoid the creditors. Her resourceful mother worked hard to put food on the table and clothes on the children, eventually leaving her abusive husband and following her two daughters across the country after the war.

As I sift through stacks of stuff in the house, I find paragraphs or a page or two of bits and starts of the story on loose papers, on the first few pages of spiral bound notebooks, and in partially used journals, along with lists of memories to write about later. She has been writing it for three decades, losing the thread, getting distracted by the present, misplacing her latest start, starting again; a patchwork pattern repeated over and over. I gather them into one box and consider presenting them to her; then decide it might feel like evidence of her scattered brain—and messing with her stuff.

"Tell me about writing your mother's story," I say instead one day.

"I promised my mother I would write it," she says.

I suspect the promise was made after my grandmother died, Mama's way of whispering *I'm sorry* for not appreciating her mother's hard work to quilt together a life for her family.

"I thought you would write her story," she says—one more expectation she had of me that she didn't tell me about.

"I'm writing my own story," I say. "I wish you would write your story rather than your mother's."

At my urging, she resumes the project. She tells me she started taping the story years back, and we go on a massive and unsuccessful hunt for the cassette tapes. She tries writing again with the felt-tip pens on pads of paper with dark lines we got from the low vision clinic, but she can no longer write legibly nor read what she has written. She returns to the obsolete tape recorder, speaking in her quavering voice. We explore up-to-date recording technology, but she needs the familiar. I replace the machine when it breaks with one nearly like it from Radio Shack just before they go out of business.

She becomes increasingly frantic to complete the project. She says she can't think of the right words anymore, and that she's forgetting the details and the dates. She can't hear what she's already recorded, and she's afraid she repeats herself. She's in a race with total memory loss, if not with death.

I have been banned from the project in favor of Stan, who has far more patience than I and more interest in the stories so familiar to me. Adding another task to his eclectic position, he spends hours with her, while the spring yard work languishes.

Jo Ann agrees to begin the tedious task of transcribing the tapes when I refuse. My life contains enough Mama. I promise to weave the transcript into a story—someday. Her obsession is going to send us all to a premature death, but it keeps her busy and gives her purpose.

༄

After dinner tonight, Mama sleeps bent forward in the kitchen chair after she crushed her multivitamin, mixed it with applesauce, and ate it. It wasn't a good day. Stan canceled. I tried to help her get started on her tape this morning, but she insisted she taped more yesterday than is on the tape.

"It isn't possible you erased anything," I reassured her. "Maybe you were just thinking about what came next. Behind every good story is a good editor. Just get it out. I will get the words right, the sequence corrected, the repetitions deleted."

Her shoulders slumped. "Maybe it's not important, and no one cares," she said quietly.

My heart broke for her. "It is important, because it's important to you." I was sorry, then, for not embracing her project with more enthusiasm. Like Russian nesting dolls, inside me is my mother, and inside her is her mother, and inside her mother is *her* mother—dead before my grandmother's age hit double digits. Our history is locked inside of us, and telling her mother's story *is* telling her own story.

A few months from now, though all the tapes aren't transcribed and Mama hasn't finished telling the story, I drop my own writing to make a comprehensible story of Mama's scrambled recording. I have it printed and bound and we present it to her on Christmas; a good faith promise that we will finish her project, continuing her own promise to her mother unto the next generation. When Rebecca reads it to her, she says I changed the story.

I watch her for a few moments now. She looks so old, so weary, so alone; so much like her mother near the end of her life. My chest tightens until I can hardly breathe. No matter how many people are around, the end of life is traveled alone. I want to pull her onto my lap, fold my arms around her tiny body and hold her to my bosom, like she once held me when I skinned my knee. I want to tell her it's okay to be sad. I want to tell her I'm sorry. Sorry she has to still be alive and not really living. Tell her she can stop working so hard to stay tethered here.

Gently waking her, I help her to bed.

55

May

Birthdays

We are baby-waiting and it's past the due date. Emma and Wynne have again chosen not to know the baby's sex, seeing it as one of life's beautiful surprises, the ultimate in anticipation. But we all sense it's a boy.

When they finally go to the hospital, I head up the interstate, handing off Mama-care to Rebecca after dinner. Emma's father and stepmother have come from Virginia for this arrival, and I am designated for Elliot-care. After checking in at the hospital when I arrive in the city and finding delivery is still a ways off, I go to the house to relieve Elliot's babysitters. As I pull up to the house, Wynne calls me to tell me Emma delivered "the babe" right after I left, surprising everyone. I check in with their friends who tell me they are fine, Elliot is asleep, and to go back. I return to the opposite corner of the city, with one last prayer for a girl, knowing it's the last chance to hope for a granddaughter.

He is beautiful, of course. *Welcome to the world, Adrian Jude.* His middle name is bestowed to honor Wynne's beautiful mother who loved the Beatles and died a few weeks ago after a lengthy illness and decline, old before her time. I whisper to him that he has the best parents in the world, and the best big brother, and that his Oomi is watching over him.

The next morning I take Elliot to the hospital. Standing witness to his two-year-old self meeting his baby brother for the first time is a highlight of my life. He sits on the bed, snuggled under Emma's arm, holding Adrian's tiny fingers, the wonder of a child's discovery shining in his blue eyes.

$\sim$

When Adrian is two weeks old, they come down to introduce him to his great-grandmother. There are ninety-nine years and eleven months difference in their ages. As my mother holds her fourth great-grandchild, I consider the differences in the worlds they were born into. Born poor when only the wealthy had a telephone and electricity, my mother's family had neither during her childhood. Adrian's mothers and I each have a smart phone in our pocket, and our homes have high-speed internet. Born before women had the right to vote, in a few months Mama will be thrilled to cast her presidential vote for Hillary Clinton. My mother's grandmothers died decades before she was born, and now advanced medical knowledge has increased life expectancy—and particularly her life—and brought the opportunity for her to know these tiny people.

Adrian rests his tiny smooth hand in his great-grandmother's gnarled one as they look into each other's eyes, and my heart bursts.

$\sim$

After Adrian's birth, I turn my full attention to the next big thing: Mama's hundredth birthday party, less than a month away. I'm beginning to understand the value of surprise birthday parties. Telling her to relax and let us take care of it doesn't help. Telling her she is making it harder on us when she tells us we are working too hard and she doesn't want people to celebrate her, doesn't help.

And besides she doesn't mean it. "If you are letting *The Today Show* know," (so she can be on the show's former weather celebrity Willard Scott's Smucker's jar), "be sure to include my maiden name in case childhood friends in Tennessee see it." Rebecca tells her they are all dead, but adds it and notification to the White House to her to-do list. Mama cannot possibly come up with anyone not on the 250-person invitation list, but she keeps asking if we invited this person and that.

Over the next weeks, I touch nearly every unsorted, unlabeled photograph in the house at least twice, choosing a representative sample of a hundred years of living, scanning and printing them, mounting them on foam board.

"There aren't going to be pictures, are there?" Mama asks one day.

"There are!" I say.

"People usually do that for a funeral."

"There won't be anyone left alive to see them by the time you die."

"You are going to too much trouble. Did you find the one of me on Mt. Pisgah? How about the one. . . ?"

I walk away.

⁓

Every day she has something new to say about the event she doesn't want but will not let us be in charge of.

"The women of the church can bring food," she says this morning.

"Mother!" I say, my nerves frayed, "we are taking care of everything! Can you just let us?"

"I don't want speeches," she says.

"There don't have to be speeches. One of us will thank people for coming and for being part of your life, and that's it. No eulogy." She starts stressing over her speech, which Rebecca helps her with. I guess it's her party. And I'll cry if I want to.

56

June

Exit Plan

For a few days after the event, Mama basks in the glow of being celebrated by friends and family, including her four great-grandsons. She's happy, sleeping well, zipping around the house without her walker, complimentary about dinner, kind to Michelle with whom she had become snippy, critical, and demanding again in recent months. Even her handwriting is less wavery as she writes thank you notes. "Who knew turning a hundred could be so much fun?" she exclaims, as I read her the more than one hundred cards, notes, and letters from her fans thanking her for what she has meant in their lives, for being the woman I wished I had known—or maybe the mother I pushed away. We never heard from the *Today Show*, but she gets a card from Michelle and Barack Obama, which pleases her.

On the sixth day after the party, seven hours after Nicholas's family left to return to North Carolina and it's back to the two of us, Mama drags hunched over her walker into the kitchen from her nap as I'm cooking dinner. "What are we having to eat?" she asks.

"I guess I can eat that," she says when I tell her.

"I want my plate hot."

"I have a cup over here."

"Heat my water for ninety seconds."

"I need Miralax in my water."

"The chard is overcooked."

"The peas have too much salt."

"My belly is upset."

"I need you to make an appointment with my doctor."

My shoulders sag; my chest resumes its familiar tightness. Mama begins telling people the day wore her out, that it was too much.

∼

A few days later, I'm sitting at my campsite in the Olympic National Park celebrating my own birthday in blessed solitude. I watch a mother duck and her two ducklings playing in the Skokomish River. The children are misbehaving, and Mama duck cackles at them, forcing them into compliance before they head downriver and join three more ducklings—the good children, I presume. I can hear them muttering, *I'll do it because I want to, not because you told me to.*

I'm tired of being cackled at by my mother. I am not a child; I shouldn't have to comply or conform. And at sixty-four I should be beyond the temptation of my own childhood mutterings and their false power.

I stare at the water as it slams into a small boulder in the river. It diverts around one side into an eddy where it's forced back against the current and around the upriver side of the rock, then set free to flow down the other side. I am water falling into a whirlpool, swirling around and around, unable to get back to freedom, too often battling upstream using hurtful words against my mother in an attempt to save myself.

It's time for an exit plan. They are the same words I heard nine years ago sitting in the porch swing of my rented house, when I formed a vague plan for my future. It made me feel more in control of my life, less like it was in control of me.

When I began that move from North Carolina four years ago, I made Rebecca promise not to let me get stuck in this house, in this town, in endless mother-care. "No matter what I say, ignore my words!" She pinky swore! She probably made the same promise to herself upon her own return. How did this town and our mother suck us back and swallow us whole?

I sip my glass of wine as the sun sinks behind the Olympics. I watch the water slam, divert, eddy, and flow free over and over. In a year I will be sixty-five, and I'll have been caring for my mother for five years—a respectable time. A pretty damn good amount of time. Could I make a change in a year? Rebecca moved on to new ventures after five years with Mama, while continuing nonresidential care. Jo Ann, at sixty-nine, has just gotten the job she's been dreaming of for over a decade. Don't I have the right to a new life too? *I promised Mama and my sisters one year. It was only to myself I later promised "till death do us part,"* I think, trying to justify the anticipation of feeling like I'm abandoning her, that I'll feel I've failed again at staying in relationship.

I've been good at protecting my need for self-care these four years, feeling no hesitation to ask my sisters to step in so I can get away. Mama has been supportive of my absences, if not about my asking Rebecca and Jo Ann to interrupt their "busy lives." But they have all been counting on me being here, shutting their eyes to the possibility that I might leave at any time, taking my presence for granted. Extraction will not be like quitting a job. I don't care; no one is going to take care of me except me.

Yes, I think, nodding to myself, *I could make a change in a year.* I don't need to know right now what will happen, only that something will change. What it will look like depends on what happens to Mama in her 101st year. It may be as simple as my taking control of the house, which will not be simple at all. If she requires a great deal more care, it may mean moving her, or leaving myself and hiring full-time care. All options will require her to adapt when she may be beyond the ability to do so, and it could hasten her downward spiral. Will it be seen as my fault? I have been a participant in keeping Mama alive beyond what even she is comfortable with, as surely as installing a pacemaker in the body of someone better served being allowed to let go of this life.

It feels like the divorce I swore wouldn't happen this time; that this time I would get it right. But there it is, I'm leaving. Again.

I feel set free.

year five

57

July

Leaving, Not Gone

When I return from my camping trip, Rebecca and I go out for dinner. "I have something to tell you," I say as she looks at me expectantly. I know I need to say it, or I will chicken out. My stomach hurts. "I've decided I need an end date for Mama-care and it needs to be by this time next year and I don't know what that will look like but it needs to be different than it is." I don't know when to take a breath. I want to crawl under the table, but I sit up tall.

"Well, anything could happen in a year," Rebecca finally says.

"I'm pretty sure she'll still be alive," I say.

"We'll figure it out," she says.

That's it? I don't know what I expected, but I feel like I need something more than "we'll figure it out." But then I've changed my mind about how long I was going to stay so many times, why should anyone believe me now?

"Should we tell Mama?" I ask.

"It doesn't seem necessary," she says. "She'll just obsess over it."

In hindsight, that might have been misguided; maybe she would have just insisted on moving right then and it would have felt like her decision. But I agree and nothing more is said.

I send Jo Ann an email and tell her my decision. She doesn't respond.

∽

I continue to do battle with my conscience. On my wedding day, I vowed to stay in my marriage until a funeral. I never considered what would come in between. I entered a relationship with a woman, not with a wedding quite—they weren't lawful in the 1990s—but with promises in front of witnesses. The relationship ended after ten years. I had become the bad girl—the woman who couldn't keep a commitment—and I didn't feel like the self I thought I was.

This time is different, I tell myself: *I'm not leaving.* I'm forging a new relationship as the participants change. It's time to turn off the tape that plays on continuous loop in my head, telling me I'm a relationship failure, that I never follow through on anything.

When I moved here I committed to being a companion, not a paid employee. Avoiding that relationship was brilliant. Of course I had no idea Mama thought I was coming so she could take care of me, that she was doing me a huge favor and therefore I would have no rights. With a click of insight, I realize the mistake I did make. Like children who take over the family farm while their parents are still alive, we should have had an understanding that we were joining our households and what that would need to look like for each of us. Those agreements should have been renegotiated each year as I committed to a longer sojourn with Mama, and as she became less able to care for her needs. I feared writing a "contract" would prevent the peer relationship I longed for with her; but instead avoidance of the conversation invited her to stay in our mother and child relationship, with opportunities for conflict.

❧

Several nights after my disclosure to Rebecca, sitting at the dining table with Mama, I'm overcome with longing. It's a beautiful evening. I want to be sitting on the deck with my dinner. Instead the glass door is closed, latched, and bolted; not a breath of air moves in the closed up room the heat pump has been chugging warmth into all day. The shades are closed against the bright light that hurts Mama's eyes. I am hemmed in, trapped in my mother's web of need and control. *Twelve months*, I tell myself, and take a deep breath, forcefully expelling it through my mouth. My sisters may not be taking me seriously, but I am.

58

August

Another Crisis

We're back in the hospital again, waiting for Mama to poop. I called Rebecca to come last evening. It was a rough night, Mama in agony and Rebecca and I wanting to avoid the hospital, missing the hospice call line. We gave in, calling the ambulance to transport her, then sat in the ER cubicle bowed over our knees, head in hands, not believing we were here again. The X-ray showed a bowel obstruction. We had made the right decision, which was small consolation.

Mama is resting "comfortably" now with a nasogastric tube up her nose, which is not comfortable. She survived its insertion, screaming in pain while Rebecca and I held each other and sobbed. I know pretty much everything about that particular torture device now, and I have increased my knowledge of abdominal anatomy.

Rebecca or I are camped out in her room twenty-four hours a day. We are being overprotective, safeguarding ourselves, as much as Mama, against ongoing fallout from imagined hospital errors when we go home.

Emma and Wynne and the little guys come for a visit. I nurture and enjoy them in my home without having to think about Mama's presence and needs while Rebecca is on duty. I don't want her to be sick and uncomfortable. I want her to come back to her familiar space. And I don't.

~

Mama finally has success in the bathroom, as she calls it. After eight days, I'm ready to be done with the hospital, but I will miss that call button, the one I'm not on the other end of. Preparing to leave, we get the bad news: we are denied a referral to hospice care by the hospital liaison. Both of the hospitalists are outraged. They give us a referral for home health, but when I call they tell me they may not get to us for a week.

Rebecca spends the first night home at the house so I can recover from the last sleepless night in the hospital. I move the monitor receiver to the guest room for her.

"Call me when you need to go to the bathroom," Rebecca tells her.

"I don't want to bother you," Mama says. "You need your sleep."

"You've been in the hospital for more than a week without much exercise or food," Rebecca reminds her. "We would rather help until you get your strength back than have you fall and need help for longer."

She gets up twice during the night without calling, Rebecca hearing her in the bathroom and getting up to assist.

"Why didn't you call?" I ask her the next morning.

"I'm fine," Mama says. "I didn't want to bother Rebecca."

"After I realized you weren't going to call, I lay awake listening for you," Rebecca chides her. "I got less sleep than if you'd called for help!"

Mama doesn't respond.

After Rebecca leaves for the day, I ask her twice if she's ready to get up for breakfast.

"I need to rest some more," she says. "Michelle can fix it when she gets here."

"She's pissed off because we 'scolded' her," I text Rebecca.

When Michelle has come and gone, Mama tells me she isn't hungry and only wants Boost for lunch. Rebecca arrives for dinner, and Mama tells her she's starving, that she didn't have breakfast until ten when Michelle made hot cereal because I wouldn't fix it for her. And, she says, she didn't have any lunch. I catch Rebecca's eye and lift mine heavenward.

༼

The next evening, my turn to cook, I hear "Grehhhhtchuuunnn" from the bedroom. It's the fourth time in twenty minutes while I'm trying to cook dinner. She has refused all day to leave her bedroom except during the two hours Michelle was with her.

"My ankles are so swollen!" she exclaims this time. "And they are painful on the top. Massage them with lotion." When I do, she shrieks, "Owoooo! Not on the top!"

"There's cold air blowing on me from the register!"

"Someone moved my comforter, and I can't reach it."

"I can't get warm. Michelle must have turned down the thermostat." I heard her tell Michelle to turn the baseboard heat down. It's eighty-five degrees in her room according to the indicator on the baby monitor.

"I need something to drink. Last night I could get it myself, but now I can't."

"Why is that?" I ask with false sweetness, engaging for the first time.

"Because you told me not to sit up."

"I did not!" I exclaim with no trace of sweet.

"You told me not to get up in the night."

I sigh and shake my head in exasperation. I know she understands the reason we told her not to get up alone, and I don't bother to correct her; she's not looking for explanation or conversation.

When I return to the kitchen, I open the freezer door. There is the pint of Snoqualmie chocolate chip mint ice cream, beckoning. I lean against the counter and start spooning it from carton to mouth, dinner preparation forgotten. "Grehhhhtchuuunnn." I sigh, return the carton to the freezer, and drag down the hall.

"I need to get into home health. I don't want you to tell them not to come. I don't want you to tell them there's no hurry."

This is the second time in twenty-four hours she has said this. I have no idea where she got the notion we were discouraging the referral. Does she think I'm insane?

"I'm not discouraging them. As a matter of fact, I just called them since they hadn't called me yet."

"I need to go to the bathroom," she says, ignoring my response. I help her stand up and get to her walker then tell her I'm going back to the kitchen.

"Should I let you know when I need to get off the toilet or do it myself?"

"You can do it yourself."

"What if I need help?" she snips. I tap my thumb and middle finger together in the Shuni Mudra I learned in yoga, to remind me to breathe and not speak until helpful words form in my head.

"Then call me to help," I say with a calm I definitely don't feel.

"You told me not to do anything myself."

My tools become shards of ineffectiveness. "No, I didn't! You are being ridiculous!"

Rebecca arrives after supper, and I head to Seattle and my little guys and their moms. Two-year-old behavior, difficult as it is, is somehow more tolerable in an actual two-year-old.

◦∼◦

It's week one of my Gigi nanny job with baby Adrian. It's been fourteen months since my year with his big brother ended. Last week, trying to help two-year-old Elliot with the concept that I am his mommy's mommy, Emma texted me a quote from him: "You no have Gigi first, Mommy! I have Gigi first!" I grab onto the lifeline of regular time with these little guys and their moms again, and I know it will be exhausting. Mama was much more independent when I cared for Elliot.

At four thirty the morning after my arrival, Elliot bounces out of bed and scampers into the living room of the tiny house where I'm sleeping on the air bed, to stand breathing next to my head. According to the moms, he was up several times during the night, alternating with the baby. I heard nothing, I was that tired.

Rebecca calls at eight o'clock to tell me Mama was wailing in pain during the night, and at six Rebecca had contacted the doctor on call, who confirmed Mama did not have any symptoms of the heart attack she was sure she was having. I want to put a pillow over my head and leave it there.

While Adrian takes a morning nap, I call Mama's doctor about her hospital follow-up appointment, respond to a recorded survey about her hospital internment, call home health (again), reschedule her dentist appointment, refer the follow-up call about Rebecca's after-hours doctor call back to Rebecca, fill out a jury duty exemption form. And I call the hospital about the flight insurance reimbursement claim the hospitalist filled out for me for my canceled trip to North Carolina to see Nicholas and Kristy and my grandsons and attend a friend's wedding that I'd been looking forward to for months. I'm long past tears.

I return home the second night, not at all sorry that traffic is heavy and it takes an hour longer than it should. I'm upstairs in the guest room for overnight bathroom duty; I barely sleep.

I'm tired, and I don't want to do this anymore. I've been here 1,506 days. I don't think I'll last the one more year.

59

September

Caregiver Hell

To prove she is still capable, when Mama recovers from the hospital stay, she and Michelle go out on errands. Mama doesn't take to her uppity daughter telling her it's too much, so I keep quiet when I see her long list. If her own poor judgment kills her, so be it. I hope it doesn't kill me and Rebecca first.

"I don't feel well," she tells me the next day. "I need more help. I need someone who is trained to work with the blind."

Rebecca and I have asked many times what that means to her. She can't answer, but she doesn't stop saying she needs it. I repeat what we always tell her: "People trained to work with the visually impaired are teaching them to use technology and walk independently with a cane or with a dog. You need someone trained to work with the elderly, and you have that. Even better, Michelle has been trained by you!"

"Michelle makes a lot of mistakes," she says.

I close my eyes and pray for mercy.

Though she can't say it, I know she wants someone who will be constantly by her side to do her bidding. We both know it's not going to be me. We need to get serious about finding her a new home and getting on a waiting list. Disaster is going to strike, and this pieced-together arrangement is not going to suffice. For now I start looking for additional hours of in-home care.

We interview another Jill, which might be a strike against her. She's a tiny woman, maybe five feet, barely as tall as Mama. I talk to her first.

"My mother will ask you if you cook," I tell her. "That will not necessarily be a function of your job, other than maybe soup."

Mama joins us and I introduce them. "Do you cook?" Mama asks immediately. "I need someone to cook dinner." I blanch. I didn't see that coming.

"Are you firing me?" I ask. I would be thrilled, but it's ludicrous.

Ignoring me, she continues talking to Jill. "I like fresh chicken baked in the oven or maybe the crock pot, and meatloaf. If you call ahead, the meat market will have fresh ground sirloin."

I keep my mouth shut. It's her interview. I don't let her choose the menu and instruct me in preparing it. I have robbed her of her superpower.

"I'm not much of a cook," Jill admits, in her lilting New Zealand accent that I know Mama will have trouble understanding.

"Do you like to make soup?" Mama asks.

"I do!" Jill says, grimacing in my direction.

❧

We hire Jill for a few hours a week. I try to let Mama help decide when Jill should arrive on her work days. As she sits across the dining table from me counting hours on her fingers and asking clarifying questions over and over, I can see on her face she is completely muddled.

"Would you like me to make the decision?" I ask gently.

"My brain seems to be worn out," she says, close to tears.

"It's been working hard for you for a long time," I say. "It's okay to accept help."

I can tell she isn't buying it, but she lets me set the hours.

We change Michelle's arrival so she can get Mama's breakfast for her, since I'm in Seattle on Michelle's days. The first day with the new schedule, she tells me she couldn't eat Michelle's first attempt at Malt-o-Meal and she wants to go back to my measuring it the night before and her cooking it, which wasn't working. After holding back my frustration, it bursts through the dam. Instead of listening behind the words, understanding that she doesn't like to give up on herself, I shout at her that she needs to give Michelle a chance. I don't think I used the "f" word.

"Well, they changed how they make Malt-o-Meal with maple and brown sugar," she says.

"You've been eating it for months," I say. "Did you get a new box?"

"No, but it's too sweet."

Like sugarplum fairies came in the middle of the night and added sugar to the half-used box.

Her taste buds are shot. Her memory knows how things used to taste—accurate or not—and nothing measures up. I'm sad for her. She is so sure there is a perfect caregiver out there—one who can cook and make her happy. I know it's dementia, and if she understood that too, maybe I could be more compassionate. I feel like my soul is being sucked out of me.

60

September

The Big One

Mama is desperately trying to hang onto memory, not realizing how much she forgets. It's maddening as she blames others for her deteriorating brain. "I try to help Michelle with her forgetfulness," she sighed the other day, after falsely accusing her of an infraction, "but I'm afraid it's a lost cause." With another mother we both would have laughed at the absurdity of the statement. This morning in Seattle, as I sit holding my sleeping grandson, I suddenly feel heart deep the shift in the mother who once held the infant me. What could be funny with acceptance is tragic instead. Like the Chutes and Ladders game I play with Elliot, Mama has landed on the square at the top of the long chute. And she's about to go over the lip.

◠

Michelle called as I put Adrian in his crib, to tell me Mama wasn't feeling well and had gone to bed. I'm on edge all afternoon, waiting for the shoe to drop. As we are finishing dinner, Rebecca calls to fling it out.

"It doesn't look good," she says.

"Shit. Should I come home?"

"Can you?" she asks.

I leave Emma and Wynne to figure out a last-minute plan for Adrian's care the next day, and drive back down I-5. Rebecca calls to say Mama is vomiting and she's called for an ambulance. *Dammit, dammit, dammit.*

The X-ray shows another blockage. "It's the way of these things," the doctor tells us, "and it will keep happening." Our options are the NG tube or wait it out and see if it clears itself. If it doesn't, she will die. She's ready to die; this may be opportunity rather than crisis. But we need hospice to help us make the decision when the time comes and to keep her comfortable. We opt for the tube again.

The blockage clears quickly this time, and she stays only two days. The hospitalist, like the two from our visit two weeks ago, thinks she should be on hospice care for recurring obstructions. *Duh.* He pushes the hospital's screening liaison to make the referral.

An hour after our return home, the hospice doctor comes to the house for an intake interview. She writes up the paperwork, and just like that, Mama is back in. I'm ecstatic.

We hadn't had time to act on our intention to start looking for a place for Mama to move to; or maybe we were stalling, thinking we were good for a while with more help at home. While we sat in the ER, Rebecca and I recommitted to beginning the search. Now we have the hospice nurse and social worker to help us.

∽

The night after our return from the hospital and our reinstated hospice status, Mama is stronger following discharge than she was two weeks earlier. Rebecca, who took the last night at the hospital, goes home after dinner, and we decide I can sleep downstairs in my own bed. Mama promises to call if she needs me.

I leave her sitting on the edge of her bed ready to lie down. I'm settling into bed with a book, Smudge on my legs, when I hear the thud and Mama's scream.

I grab my phone and race upstairs, trying to get Siri to dial Rebecca as I take the steps two at a time, but Siri can't understand my panicked voice prompt. Mama is lying face down in the hallway, her right arm folded under her, and she is hysterical. I call hospice, the first line of defense, then 911 as instructed.

I speak to Mama calmly as I gently turn her onto her side to free her arm. She moans in pain. The mug of microwaved water she had apparently gone to the kitchen to get is on the carpet and she's lying in a puddle. She's cold. I get pillows, cover her with multiple blankets, and soak up what water I can with a towel. I stroke her head while we wait for Rebecca and the EMTs.

◠◡

X-rays in the ER show breaks in the wrist and shoulder of her dominant arm.

"How did you fall?" the ER doctor asks.

"I don't know what happened." She sounds muddled. "My shoes stick to the rug sometimes. I must have tripped."

I look at Rebecca, shaking my head. "She didn't have her shoes on," I whisper.

Rebecca's eyes widen. She never leaves her room without putting on her shoes.

"Was my walker in the hall, Gretchen?"

"No," I say; "it was in the bedroom. I think you had something in each hand, so you couldn't hold onto the wall either."

She doesn't say anything more. I wonder if she believes me.

Later she tells people she got cocky and did a "stupid, stupid thing," for once taking responsibility. Cocky or not, the lapse in judgment is not like her.

The slogan on the computer screen savers at the Sisters of Providence hospital is becoming permanently inscribed on my brain: "All that I know of tomorrow is that Providence will rise before the sun."

All I know of weeks of tomorrows is that they're going to be hell.

∽

We are in a different country now. Mama can't walk, toilet, or eat by herself. She can't get in and out of bed or a chair without heavy lifting on someone's part. She can't even move in bed without help. She is on a triad of bowel aids that have to be administered by someone to be sure she takes them. There are many trips to the bathroom. This is 24-hour care.

For the most part, she has been uncharacteristically brave and pleasant. It's amazing the difference that makes for me.

As promised, we get the same hospice team. When Laurel comes today, I hug her like the life preserver she is.

"It will get more painful," she says.

"Do you mean for Mama or for me?" I ask.

"Both," she chuckles. "We're here with you, though."

"Stella," she says before she leaves, "you need to take the half tablets of pain medication. Gretchen will give them to you on a schedule. Don't fight her!"

"Okay," Mama says.

After lunch, I give her the tablet.

"I don't need it," she says. "I don't like to take medication."

"You have to take it," I say. "You promised Laurel." She sighs and holds out her hand for it and I watch her swallow it. I'm fighting for my life too.

~

Elliot calls me on FaceTime the day before my next trip up I-5: "Gigi! Bring more apples! Gigi's apples!" he shouts. My little boys will get me through this, and I will not give up my time with them.

61

September

Liminal Space

It's autumn, that liminal Pacific Northwest season when the days hopscotch from overcast and rainy and the quiet of winter seems around the corner, to blue skies and warm sun and it feels as if extrovert summer will go on and on.

Mama is in liminal space too, holding me and Rebecca there with her. She teeters on the threshold between the familiar problems and the new, between life and maybe the end. I feel on the brink of new life for me but not yet free to step into it.

It's been pleasurable to care for her the past couple days, to help her be comfortable, to encourage her to try new things like eating with her left hand, which she quickly masters—her stubborn persistence paying off. She continues to be kind and grateful, brave and uncomplaining. She asks for what she needs without a hint of whine. Following a long nap today—part of what made the day pleasurable for both of us—she tells me her dream. "I was in Alaska and couldn't see anything. It was grey above and icy below. And I couldn't find anything to eat."

My eyes fill. "That sounds frightening," I say.

～

Rebecca misses the first day of the weekend Portland Market, an annual buying trip for her shop. Mama has been so easy, I insist she go for the second day and put together a seamless caregiving schedule for the days I'll be in Seattle, using temporary help from the agency Michelle works for, along with Michelle and Jill.

By midmorning on Sunday, after Rebecca's early departure, Mama is spinning downward at a dizzying pace. I can't do anything right, and her constant demands give me ample opportunity to fail. I was in her room more than mine last night, and when she sleeps today, I sleep. The latch on the garden gate doesn't get fixed and the deer enjoy the tomatoes, chard, peppers, and squash blossoms, and a romp in the strawberry patch. Paid work doesn't get done. I give up any hope of one more trip to the mountains before the snows come and cancel my registration for the local writers' conference on Saturday.

～

Mama does well with the paid help while I'm in Seattle, but then the tide shifts again. I'm preparing to head home Tuesday evening when Rebecca calls.

"When I got here to cook dinner Mama was in bed, moaning."

"Oh, god," I say.

"I called the hospice nurse. She told me to give her the antinausea-anxiety med in the hospice kit."

"Did she take it?"

"Yes, not happily. She said she should have just died when she fell."

"I'm on my way home," I sigh, hoping road construction will cause a significant delay.

I wonder if thinking it was the end is why she had been so patient and gracious, until she realized she wasn't going anywhere. Rebecca and I have both been encouraged by friends whose parent has been on this threshold not to be afraid to tell her it's okay to let go. As I drive down I-5, the three-quarter moon hanging over pink-bathed Mt. Rainier, I chant into the setting sun: "It's okay to let go, it's okay to let go."

"You've had a long life," Rebecca is telling Mama at the same time, "it's okay to let it go now." When she tells me later, and we realize we were entreating her at the same time, she says Mama had been quiet, then asked, "Is the window open?"

She'd slept then, but is awake and agitated again when I get home at eight thirty. We call the hospice nurse to come, and I read Mary Oliver poems to her while we wait.

The nurse determines from bowel tones that there is no obstruction. She gives her a sleep med and then leaves. It's eleven thirty. I hear Mama and Rebecca up once in the bathroom a few hours later. She's still sleeping in the morning when we leave her with Michelle, Rebecca to go home to get ready for work, me to a coffee shop to breathe for a while—a downtown one, rather than my usual one in Olympia. It's been four weeks since I went to yoga.

Maybe she is waiting for Jo Ann to come; she is trying to clear her schedule. Maybe if she sees her great-grandchildren once more; they will come next weekend. She seems to be teetering but doesn't know how to give up, to take the big step. She told the hospice doctor that yes, she would go back to the hospital for another agonizing and invasive intubation if she has another obstruction. *Why?* She tells me she needs her multi-vitamin. *Why?* She eats even though she doesn't feel like it. *Why?* She has said in the past she wants to be here as long as she can walk and see the hills. Both have been taken from her.

∽

There might as well be an electronic monitor on my ankle; I can only be as far away from Mama as her voice will reach unless someone else is with her. I entertain myself by reorganizing the kitchen while Mama takes long naps and isn't available to tell me not to. I clean out two drawers, throwing out the paper doilies that have languished there since circa 1968 and brittle roasting bags in a faded box from before the age of code scanners. There is sand in the back of what used to be "the bread drawer." Nicholas and Emma came for solo visits every summer—flying alone across the country. "I always missed them when they left," Mama has told me. "Then I would open the bread drawer and find rocks and fir cones they had hidden there, reminders." Apparently she left their residue to drift to the back corners. My chest is tight as I wipe it out. Those days are so far in the past. And I miss my own far away grandchildren.

Another day I tackle the cabinet over the refrigerator holding cold cereal boxes, most of which no one who lives here eats and will be stale by the time occasional guests return. I haven't eaten cold cereal since I outgrew Cocoa Krispies. Holding an over-sized boat-shaped salad bowl that is full of paper products and plastic cutlery lofted to the back of the cabinet, I twirl back into the past.

I'm standing on the edge of the side lawn in my nightgown, like some modern day Scrooge. It's 1969 and my parents are hosting a luau-themed party for summer interns from my father's office. Neil Armstrong and Buzz Aldrin are walking on the moon, and everyone looks up at the waxing crescent. The black wooden bowl, filled with fruit salad, sits on the long plywood and sawhorse table. My father is tending a fire in the pit, grilling king salmon and turning foil-wrapped sweet corn in the coals. I look for my mother in the crowd and don't see her. She's probably in the kitchen where she was most content.

Though my mother liked to provide, she was not comfortable in social situations. When my father became "the boss," she stepped up to her role of entertaining his colleagues and visiting dignitaries, seeing it as her responsibility to his work, like doing her part in the war effort in the 1940s and her activism in later years. It wasn't until he died in 2009 that I realized Norman Borlaug, father of the Green Revolution and 1970 Nobel Prize winner, had once sat at our dining room table, no doubt eating my mother's stuffed salmon, under-the-sea Jell-O salad, and blackberry pie. In spite of her introversion, she has always done what needed to be done.

I stuff the bowl into the cabinet in the basement and move on to the bathroom drawer while Mama sleeps on, holding me within shouting range when she wakes to go to the bathroom.

We three girls used one sink in the Jack and Jill bathroom—that mid-century innovation of separate sink areas with one tub between—sharing one drawer. I throw out the perfume and lipstick samples from Frederick and Nelson—my mother's favorite Seattle department store, which went out of business in 1992. The dried out individual packets of Wet Ones remind me of those passed from my mother's purse to us three girls in the back seat of the '56 Chevy station wagon on road trips, followed by a half stick of Juicy Fruit gum for each of us. I can still feel their peppery lemonyness tickling my nose. I wonder if the Smithsonian would like the sanitary belt, dating from before pads had sticky backs and before my mother let me wear tampons, not knowing Jo Ann had taught me to use them my sixteenth summer. The cabinet that once stored Kotex napkins and Tampax tampons now holds baby wipes, incontinence briefs, and chucks pads to protect the mattress. I remove years-old prescriptions from the cabinet on Mama's side of the bathroom and leave the tubes of red and deep pink lipstick on the shelf, proof that she was once younger.

∽

Bedtime takes a full hour, from teeth cleaning to lights out. Mama's not ready to start the process until I'm ready to be in bed. My escape downstairs after dinner, leaving her to get herself ready for bed, with twelve delicious hours to myself, is a distant memory. I hand her first the large and then the small between-the-teeth brushes, followed by whichever regular brush she requests with or without toothpaste, then a flossing stick, all used with her left hand. Next is toileting and heating rice bags to exactly the right temperature, which I never get right. I remove her hearing aid, administer eye drops, adjust her splint, and attempt to get the bed covers just right. Then she wants to sit up for more water and has to be resettled. I shudder to think of the time added should she resume getting dressed in the morning, adding undressing to the evening routine.

By the time she's satisfied, my stomach is in a knot from trying not to scream at her in frustration. I fall into bed, where I listen to her mumble in her sleep on the monitor, finally falling asleep myself before I hear "Greeetchuuun"—a name I'm beginning to loathe—and go upstairs to take her to the bathroom and settled into bed again. Back downstairs, I lie awake the rest of the night, trying not to break into tiny pieces.

62

October

Considering Options

I can't do this for the eight more months I told my sisters I would. I'm bone-tired. I want to be a daughter again, and there is no time for that. It's impossible to hold good memories, or listen to Mama's stories, or even read to her when I'm exhausted by the person she is now. David told me in our last session, three months ago, "a fall will change everything." And so it has. Maybe this is a temporary setback, but I don't think she will walk independently again. If her bones heal, I fear she will have lost all strength. But I have learned not to underestimate her.

∾

"Maybe I should stop eating and wither away," she says over dinner tonight.

"Can you say more about that?" I ask, neither encouraging nor discouraging the line of thinking.

"I'm ruining your lives, and it's not good for me either."

"Do you worry about what will happen to me when you're gone?" I've wondered if this is what keeps her bound to life.

"I worry about all of you when I'm gone," she corrects. She's never willing to single out one daughter as the focus of her attention. But without job or partner, I think I'm the one she most believes must be unhappy.

"What do you worry about?" I ask.

"That things won't turn out the way you expect them to."

"Have things always turned out the way I expected in the past?"

"No, I guess they haven't."

"And how did I do with it in the past?"

"Pretty well, I guess."

"Yes, pretty well. And have things always turned out for you the way you expected?"

"No."

"And you have done really well. It's hard, and then we figure it out and keep going, and often it's better than we'd imagined. You have been an amazing role model in how to overcome adversity and keep going. You are my inspiration."

There's a long silence and I think the conversation is over. Then she says, "Well, thank you for saying that."

A few minutes later she asks me to crush her multi-vitamin and mix it with a teaspoon of water and a teaspoon of applesauce. I have inadvertently boosted her will to live.

∽

Sunday is a beautiful autumn day. I ask Mama twice if she wants to sit on the deck and breathe the Pacific Northwest air. "No," she says, simply.

She tells Laurel she is depressed and repeats that she wishes she had died when she fell. The fact is, we all wish she had died rather than face her dismal future. It horrifies and angers me that people facing rapid decline and a life without living must linger on with little recourse unless they have a terminal illness for which they can stop treatment.

I make soup for her, make sure she takes her bowel meds, attempt to make her and her broken arm comfortable, and wipe her butt—the line I said I would not cross. Other memoirists write, "My mother wiped my bottom, it's my turn to repay her," which is ludicrous. We are supposed to wipe our babies' tiny, firm bottoms. They have no concept of how to do it for themselves, nor ability, nor embarrassment for the wiper. They will learn how to do it themselves, because we will teach them. That is the natural order of things. This is not.

I'm not embarrassed as I snap on latex gloves and pull a baby wipe out of the box. It's not that I'm squeamish as I gently search through the soft folds of skin that hang from her bony frame while she bends over her walker, looking for the feces hiding there that will cause her skin to break down and sores to form if not cleaned. I'm not resentful that I must do this task. Well, maybe a little; I don't want this to be our relationship. Mostly I'm sad. She should not be subjected to this indignity. She should be able to cling to the memory of the love with which she cared for her helpless babies. How dare this beautiful strong body betray my beautiful strong mother. How dare it.

❧

Rebecca and I have said when Mama needed twenty-four-hour care, it would be time to find her a new home, no more waffling. I talk to my sisters. We are in agreement: we can't sustain care the way we have been doing it. Two hospitalizations and a fall in a single month have, if nothing else, made us aware of what is inevitably coming as she steps back from a final decline on some days and returns to the edge on others.

But it's one thing to say we can't do this and another to stop doing it. Rebecca and I find ourselves stepping to the edge of justifying radical change and then backing off. We tell ourselves it's okay—even crucial—to take care of ourselves first. We know she doesn't want us to sacrifice our own health and happiness for hers, even as she asks us to do just that, but we avoid the conversation with her. We have dropped some hints and hope it won't come as a shock to her when we finally tell her. I dread it, but maybe she is waiting for us to bring it up.

Today, sitting with her at breakfast, Mama tells me we need to get more help or she needs to die. I wonder if she means she doesn't want Rebecca and me to have to fill this role, or that we are doing it poorly. Likely some of each.

I spontaneously jump into the opening she has created.

"There is another option," I say, my stomach contents rising to my throat. "We could find a place for you to live that would provide you with more care and attention, and allow me and Rebecca just to be your daughters again."

"Maybe," she says, unusually quickly. "But not in Centralia."

"Maybe we could be a bit more optimistic," I sigh. I don't say anything more. The idea has been introduced; she needs to live with it in her head for a while. Badgering her is counterproductive. I've learned that much, at least.

೧◡

It won't be easy to monitor her care elsewhere, making sure she is having the best quality of life she can. I know Rebecca and I will be unable to leave her somewhere and not be hypervigilant—and having her thirty miles away in Olympia is not practical. But to be able to come home after visits, knowing she is being cared for, will be life-giving. I'll have time for peer relationships, to go to Seattle to watch Elliot play soccer, to attend concerts and take ukulele lessons and write and hike, to begin my dream for the property. And be my mother's daughter. Maybe I'm delusional, but I'm already starting to breathe again.

63

October

Anticipating Change, or Not

Mama calls me upstairs only once in the night to use the bathroom—and not until four o'clock—but I haven't slept well waiting for her to call me or thinking she was calling when she was muttering in her sleep. I can't get her comfortable once she is back in bed, and the response to her call takes forty-seven minutes.

I drift back to sleep and dream. *Two young deer—"friends" of mine—are crossing the interstate. I pull to the center median and get out of my car, screaming at them to get out of the road. Suddenly I look up to see a semi on fire careening wildly out of control heading straight toward me. I try in slow motion to reach my car to drive out of the truck's path.*

I wake up, shaking, the nightmare unresolved, as is the way of nightmares.

When I'm sure she's up, I text Rebecca my dream. She replies that she had lain awake thinking how bad it would be if something happened to one of us and Mama wasn't in place somewhere.

My phone rings as we're texting. It's Michelle. She woke in the middle of the night in immobilizing back pain. She can't work at this level of care and lifting. Not today, not ever.

I abandon texting and call Rebecca in shock.

"I didn't think about something happening to Michelle!" she exclaims.

"What are we going to do?" I start to cry. "I can't do this! I'm so tired."

᠔

An hour later I call Rebecca to come to the house. I'm in full meltdown after Mama called me to help her out of bed at the same moment the substitute caregiver rang the doorbell while I was trying to tell Michelle's supervisor on the phone that I couldn't deal with a new person right now, and Laurel is due soon too. I want to get back in bed and pull the covers over my head.

I'm still trying to get it together when Laurel and Rebecca arrive.

We sit at our usual places at the table as Laurel chats with Mama.

"Would you talk to her about moving?" Rebecca whispers.

"I just can't do this anymore," I whimper, my head in my hands.

Laurel jumps in without hesitation. "Your daughters are worried they can no longer keep you safe at home, Stella, and they are really tired. What are your thoughts about that? How would you feel about going somewhere that you could be cared for?"

"I worry about them too," Mama says with tears in her eyes.

Wanting her to know we aren't going to abandon her, I add, "We want to be able to be your daughters, to listen to your stories, to read to you, to share our lives with you. And to know you are being well cared for when we can't be with you." Mama doesn't say anything.

"Maybe we can find a space in an adult family home," Laurel tells her. "They are facilities in a home-like setting with four to six residents and one or two caregivers. What would you think about that?

"That would be good," Mama says. Then adds in a near whisper,

"It would be very temporary, wouldn't it?" Laurel skirts the question and Rebecca's and my hearts shatter.

Laurel pulls out her phone and calls five owners of homes she knows to be good—some of them with multiple homes—as well as a larger facility she suggests. None of the homes has an opening except the one that is our last choice because it's twenty minutes away.

"It's wonderful care, and creepy decor. French Provincial with dolls," Laurel tells us, raising her eyebrows.

I hug Laurel as she leaves, overcome with grief and gratitude. When I feel like running with scissors, I am stopped by knowing hospice is walking with me and will gently take the scissors from my hand. I have read that the original hospice was a rest house for weary pilgrims on sacred journeys. I am grateful for the company on this journey toward death.

∽

That afternoon, Rebecca and I go visit the doll house—essentially a double-wide on the prairie. We look at each other in horror. It looks like Liberace's living room. I look around for candelabras. Porcelain dolls in elaborate dress stare at us from shelves in every corner. With a solarium off the living and dining area, there is nowhere to be that the light wouldn't hurt Mama's eyes. It has no furniture suitable for sitting on anyway. The bedroom is tiny, and they ask that residents not bring their own furniture for their rooms, which is absurd.

We manage to thank the owner graciously on our way out and barely make it to the car before we explode in laughter.

"Well, that's out of the question!" Rebecca says.

"Even if she couldn't see it," I say.

I fight tears all the way home.

❧

We're back to square one, the square that contains only us and Mama and Jill, our unseasoned caregiver with few available hours.

Jill calls as I'm preparing dinner after our return from the doll house. I brace myself for more bad news, reaching for my wine glass.

"I've called Kim," she says, a caregiver we thought we had secured following our first hospital stay who had to back out, but who recommended Jill to us. "She is available again and wants to help!" Mama knows and loves Kim. I don't even try to stop the tears.

She has also found two other caregivers she knows with available hours. We interview them and choose Bonnie to join the team. I work up a forty-hour schedule for the three of them. If full days were covered during the week, could I stay in the house with Mama until an adult family home we like has a room? Of course I will have to schedule and train and keep track of hours, fill in when a caregiver is out at the last minute, and listen to Mama's inevitable complaints of their ineptness—real and imagined. And still cook dinner and get up in the middle of the night and be confined to home evenings and weekends. It won't be a solution for long.

❧

I have been drawing a single card from my tarot deck each morning while Mama sleeps, and meditating on it as a tool to understand my life and make choices about living more fully. This morning I drew the death card. In my beautiful deck, depicting the archetypal images in detailed scenes from the natural world, there is a beached rotting rowboat that can no longer traverse the waters, but is beautiful in its grey and crumbling form. It is surrounded by the living waters, blooming flowers, a waiting vulture. Life and death side by side.

The sunrise this morning is one of the most beautiful I have seen. I sit in my chair in the corner of the living room holding the card, the baby monitor on the table beside me, and weep at the beauty of the pink-and-orange sky over the fog-filled valley, the mountain a black silhouette on the horizon. Moving Mama to a care facility feels like a giant step toward death. For the first time, I grieve the loss of my mother, even while she lives on.

64

October

Coming Unglued

We give up for now on the adult family homes and visit the seventy-resident assisted living facility Laurel suggested. They don't provide skilled nursing, but the director promises they can care for Mama for the rest of her life. We talk with Mama about it and she agrees—at least in theory.

We take her to visit. She seems impressed enough, but when the director asks if she would like to come and live with them, Mama tells her it's up to her daughters. I guess it is, and it's hard to bear the responsibility.

My mother lived in twelve homes before she graduated from high school, and nearly that many more as an adult before her current home was built. She told me her dream as a young woman was to stay put. I remind myself as we prepare her for a move that her dream was fulfilled. She has been in one home for fifty-six years. And I feel guilty.

I'm clinging on with my fingernails, and they are breaking one by one. Rebecca and hospice take the lead in all the conversations about moving while I remain intentionally in the background, since I have a conflict of interest. Still, Mama seems to blame me. The decision may have been her daughters', but she isn't going to go willingly.

◠

The past two nights, with Rebecca on overnight duty, Mama hasn't gotten up for the first time in five weeks. Today, when I send Jill home thirty minutes early—with pay—so I can have some kitchen solitude for dinner prep, I tell her not to wake Mama before she leaves, as Mama had instructed her to do after finally agreeing to nap in her bed. Jill says she's only been sleeping half an hour, but now I hear her talking clock every few minutes as she checks the time so she won't stay in bed a minute longer than the hour she'd allowed herself. Exactly thirty minutes after Jill leaves, Mama calls for her and is irate when I tell her I am responsible for her leaving early.

"This is when Jill would have left," I argue. "You're up when you wanted to be."

"I don't want to sleep during the day!" she snaps. "I want to be able to sleep at night so I don't have to bother you!"

"You've only been in bed for an hour," I say calmly, not matching her irritation, "and I wanted some quiet time in the kitchen."

"Well, then," she says in the snippy tone she has adopted only with me lately, "I won't feel bad getting you up in the night." I can't believe she said that. I help her up, take her to the bathroom, and walk her to the living room, where she sleeps soundly in her chair until dinner.

Maybe her reluctance to go to bed at night or lie down during the day, and her neediness at night—getting us up and keeping us there—are manifestations of fear of the unknown next. If this is hard for me, it's exponentially harder for her. My heart is like the battered tin colander in the cupboard, momentary understanding draining right out.

True to her threat, she calls me upstairs at top volume at one thirty in the morning.

"I kept waiting for you to come back before you went to bed to see if I wanted to go to the bathroom again," she says while I wait outside the bathroom door. "If you had, I wouldn't have had to bother you." I stick to my vow not to engage in conversation during the night, so I don't tell her I went to bed right after I got her tucked in.

Back in bed she says her fingers are swollen again, and her forearm. The swelling is greatly reduced from twenty-four hours ago, perhaps because Rebecca persuaded her to take ibuprofen every six hours as prescribed, even as Mama continued to insist it "makes her more blind."

I don't know what she expects me to do about it right now. "We aren't going to talk about it in the middle of the night," I tell her. "I can give you an ibuprofen; that's all I can do."

"I don't want to, but if that's all you'll do, I guess I will." God, I am sick of this. I cover her up, carefully arranging and rearranging the bedding, and she says, "I need a warm rice bag for my knees." I breathe deeply, choose one of the two small bags, knowing the one she used to use has been recently declared too heavy. As I leave the room to put it in the microwave, she says to my retreating back, "Heat it for three minutes." I set the timer for the usual two minutes.

"It's too hot," she complains when I return to the room and put it in place, "and I need the small one." I'm getting seriously close to tipping over the edge.

"It *is* one of the small ones," I say through clenched teeth. "I'll put it next to you and you can move it when it cools.

"I can't find it," she says. I put her hand on it. "I need my squeeze

ball," she says. I gulp air and blow it out slowly as I rummage unsuc-
cessfully through the six layers of covers for the ball—cursing that
she won't use a duvet—then go to the living room and find a different
squeeze toy.

"I can't find the ball," I tell her. "Here's the other one."

"Maybe it's in my chair in the living room," she says. Of course
the chair was the first place I had looked. Tears leak from my eyes.
I'm so tired I can hardly stand. I search the bed again, then return to
the living room and find it under the chair. I put it in her hand and
pull up the layers of covers for the third time, tucking them around
her shoulders—as I know she is about to tell me to do—and try to
anticipate which of the ever-changing specifications will come up
this time. The latest one is that none of the layers be folded over at
the top except the flannel sheet, which I have done as prescribed. As
I finish she barks at me, "I don't want any of them doubled except the
sheet!" I've been patient for forty minutes; she finally gets me.

"Why are you doing this to me?" I scream in tears of frustration.

"Who is the patient here?" she snaps.

"Well, not you!" I snap back, meaning she isn't being patient. Also
she isn't a patient, she's an old woman who has become ridiculously
needy.

"Then maybe I should be taking care of you," she says.

"Wouldn't that be nice," I say. And there it is: I want my mother
back. I want to leave the nightmare and get into bed with her and feel
warm and safe from the bad guys.

Back in my own bed, I don't bother to try to go back to sleep right
away. I hate it when I lose my temper; it proves her point that I'm a
hothead. I flip on my light and try to read until the knot in my stomach untwists. I can't concentrate on the book. I turn out the light and
watch the moon travel across the sky over the fog-filled valley and try

to remember why I moved here. A train whistle screams through the sleeping town and sets the coyotes to howling. I'm too exhausted to join the chorus.

～

Mama wakes me at seven—well past the time I usually get up—to go to the bathroom again. She wasn't aware, but she has a small mess in her incontinence pants. I clean her up and take her back to the edge of her bed, praying she won't want to get up.

"What time is it?" she asks.

"Six thirty," I tell her, though it's seven twenty. I move her clock out of reach.

"When Kim gets here, tell her to get me up. I don't want to sleep during the day and lie awake at night."

I want to ask her how that worked for her yesterday, but she wouldn't understand my sarcasm.

As I head downstairs my phone pings with a new text message. It's my cousin, telling me her ninety-eight-year-old mother has died. I am filled with envy that both my aunt and my cousin are set free from this old-age hell.

I'm dressed and ready to get to my desperately needed weekly friend date at the coffee shop. Kim is fifteen minutes late. Then thirty. I call her. She thought she was scheduled for the afternoon and says she'll be here in ten minutes.

I head to Mama's room with dread. She'll be furious she's not up. I'm glad I lied to her about the time earlier. "My legs are cold and numb," she says in response to my fake cheerful greeting. "Heat my rice bags."

"Do you want to get up?" I ask.

"First I have to get my feet warm," she says.

She's still in bed when Kim arrives and I leave the house. Walking up to the coffee shop—forty-five minutes late—Rebecca sends me a text reminding me I agreed to do something for her in an hour and wondering if she is supposed to do dinner tonight because she has no clue what to cook. I order my latte and sit down, my head on the table, crying as my friend strokes my back.

65

October

House of Mirrors

We have all come to an uneasy agreement for Mama to move to the Manor—the assisted living facility—and anticipate the move in a week and a half. I'm giddy over the change it will mean in my life. At the same time I try to put myself in my mother's place, remembering my grief as I prepared to leave my house in North Carolina, where I had lived just five years, not eleven times that. And I was ready for adventure, not waiting for death to come. I need to take care of myself, and I feel selfish. I look up selfish in the online thesaurus: self-centered, self-absorbed, self-obsessed, self-seeking, self-serving; inconsiderate, thoughtless, uncaring. The words and the feelings clog my arteries. My friends and blog readers offer encouraging words, but nothing helps. My heart hurts.

❧

A week before the move, one of the adult family homes calls. They have an opening. Rebecca and I drop everything and go to see it. We are impressed and conflicted.

It would resolve our primary concern about the larger facility: the large resident-to-caregiver ratio. We have both envisioned Mama sitting alone in her room. We worry she will think she has pushed her call button when she hasn't, and that her constant neediness will become a wolf cry as she monopolizes the time of busy aides. We wonder how she will eat meals without one-on-one attention in the dining room.

On the other hand, the available room at the AFH is small, not suitable for spending time in, and she values her privacy. The hallway, though wide, is short. Mama likes to move. The large facility has a looping hall to push the walker she may or may not be able to use again. The other AFH residents are not active. It's more a place to go to die than the Manor with its activities and broad range of levels of need.

The hospice team thinks the AFH is what she needs now as her broken arm heals and she works to regain strength. and that it's what she will continue to need as she declines. The decision, they say, shouldn't be made on a hypothetical and short-lived return to some degree of independence, and multiple transitions are not a good plan for the old-old. We are in agony. Why did we wait until we were in crisis to explore the options? We talked about the need for a plan from time to time, but subconsciously engaged in the magical thinking that it wouldn't come to this, and did nothing. Besides, getting through the present took all my energy.

გ

On Thursday, we take Mama to visit the home. She hates it and says she'll only go the Manor. Since Rebecca and I know Mama's capacity to rebound, we are in agreement.

On Saturday, she says she will only move to the AFH. The decision can't be hers, of course, but if we have learned anything over these years, it's that every decision is easier on all of us if she thinks it's her idea. Our task is to guide her to the one we have made.

Sunday she begins waffling again on moving at all.

"I could get live-in help," she tells Rebecca. She does not discuss it with me. She knows Rebecca has the softer heart and is more likely to be swayed. It's not a viable option for so many reasons, but I wait it out. I don't remind my sisters that I will move if Mama doesn't.

Monday, when I leave for Seattle in the dark, Mama has said she will move next week—to the Manor. I'm getting whiplash. While I'm away, I get reports that she told Laurel she was okay with the move—but only to the AFH. I drink a rare second glass of wine with Emma and Wynne.

I return from Seattle on Tuesday to find that Mama has miraculously—or from sheer force of will—gone from an inability to walk unassisted to using her walker independently in the thirty-six hours I've been away. *Great,* I think, *that will make the adjustment to her new home easier for all of us.* Mama views it differently. She's home free. She doesn't need to move and is back to insisting on twenty-four-hour care at home.

We have told her we'll bring her back to the house often, that at least one of us will see her every day, that her friends will visit and she'll make new friends, but she has dug in her heels. "If I don't have enough money for twenty-four-hour care at home," she tells Rebecca, "I'll sell the house to pay for it." She can't be rational; we can't expect her to be. She is scared to leave her familiar.

We all need a break. I call the director at the Manor and tell her the move-in date has been put off. She assures me the room is still available. I'm sure we are not the first family to struggle with this transition.

❧

A few days later, Jo Ann arrives for a visit, after I urged and Rebecca guilted her into it. The dates were chosen to help with a transition that's on hold. Now we hope the voice of the eldest and best-because-she-doesn't-live-here daughter will help get a decision made. Laurel comes to moderate an intervention.

Mama opens the conversation, and I know immediately she is going to try to lure us back into the rabbit hole.

"Do you know any caregivers who would live in?" she asks.

"No, I don't," Laurel says firmly, refusing to dive into her fantasy.

"There must be someone at the church who needs a place to live. They could have the guest room," Mama insists, still wanting to believe all she needs is a roommate.

"It's not an option, honey," Laurel says.

She is grasping, frantic to stay in her home she so many times in the past four years threatened to leave when things weren't going well with me. Should we have called her bluff? She isn't thinking about being one hundred years old and about what might be best for her. She is grieving the fact that she is no longer raising her family in this home, that she can no longer see the sunrise or dig in her garden or do crafts. Or take care of herself. I am caught between sorrow and exasperation.

The next morning, after a sleepless night, Mama has decided again she will go.

∽

Rebecca and I have been talking since the first hospitalization after my arrival about when we will know the home gig is up, if not about where Mama will go. And now we are here. I thought we were on the same page, but her soft heart is melting, and I sense a growing reluctance about a move.

Somewhere in the recesses of childhood memory is a trip through the House of Mirrors at some summer fair. Everywhere I turned I met myself. Those accompanying me kept changing as strangers drifted by, sometimes walking with me, other times walking into the distance. But always I was there, the constant as I tried to find my way through the maze. As I sense Rebecca's misgivings, I'm back in the mirrors. One day Rebecca is standing with me and Mama is left behind; other days she stands with Mama while I stand in the distance, fractured, lost, alone.

Mama can't understand that she is incapable of making this decision, Rebecca is loath to decide for her, Jo Ann won't take a position, and I don't want to divide myself from the family.

66

October

Scam

Despite my sense of Rebecca's unspoken uneasiness with the move, she continues to be outwardly engaged with the plan. Now it's us changing our minds every few hours about the right placement, while Jo Ann continues to express no opinion.

Jo Ann and I take Mama to see both places again. I'm hoping Jo Ann will have a fresh perspective. I leave them in the car and go into the AFH first to make sure it's a convenient time to visit. The aide tells me they have given the room to someone else. I stand next to the oversized dining table in the room that is the kitchen, dining room, and living room—where a resident stares unseeing at a soap opera on a muted TV—looking at the aide in stunned silence.

At first I'm irritated that they didn't give us first refusal; I was told they would hold it for a week. But this morning Rebecca and I had changed our minds again, leaning toward the privacy, spaciousness, and opportunities available at the larger place, so it makes the decision easier. For once Mama's preference-of-the-day is in alignment with ours; at least it was at breakfast.

"Well, the room is no longer available," I tell Mama and Jo Ann on my return to the car.

"I'm not going to visit the Manor," Mama says.

"Why is that?" I ask.

"Because I'm not going to move there."

I glance up at Jo Ann in the rearview mirror with raised eyebrows and shrug my shoulders. *You see what this has been like?*

We visit the larger facility anyway, and this time "her" room is ready to see. Jo Ann and I enthusiastically point out the ramp in the parking lot Mama insisted wasn't there, the elevator, the wide halls for walking, the alcoves for sitting, the second floor veranda on the shaded side of the building. We both notice the smell of cat pee and human urine near some of the doors we pass and my heart sinks. *How can we do this to her?*

I look at the names on all the doors looking for a familiar one. A few doors from her room is the favorite English teacher Rebecca and I had in high school and Mama is excited. "I've always wanted to know her!" she says. Jo Ann and I do a mental high five.

That evening Mama talks about the room that will be hers. I start breathing again. It's going to happen.

I should know better by now.

∽

I return from Seattle with a cold. Although I slept well on the air bed in Emma and Wynne's living room, the day began very early. After the long drive home in the rain and dark, I'm longing to fall into bed. I greet Mama who is still in the living room with Jo Ann, not started for bed, where she normally already would be at this hour. I don't have the energy to interact, but I can't avoid her.

"Hello!" I shout to be heard.

"Who's there?" she says, her usual reply. I never understand who she thinks it would be. I feel like I'm on the set of *Wait Until Dark*.

"Gretchen!" I say with a brightness I don't feel.

"I thought you weren't coming home until tomorrow." She always says that too.

"Nope," I say, wishing it were true.

"I am not moving!" she uncharacteristically shouts. "And you can't make me! This is *my* house and it's *my* money and *you* can't have it all." I didn't see that coming. My stomach bottoms out.

"I'm not taking your money," I say, glancing at Jo Ann, mouthing *what the fuck?* She shrugs and raises one eyebrow, a trick I wish I could do.

"Your daddy would be very unhappy with you!" Jo Ann and I both blanch. That is as deep a blow as she knows how to deliver. I flash back to the day of his burial when she blurted out that he had been very unhappy with me. It took a long time to heal from her words about his continuing anger over my divorce on that already difficult day and the implications about his love for me; but I have, and I'm not going back down that hole with her.

I take a calming breath, kneel beside her, and gently say what I know to be true: "I think Daddy would be very proud of me. I've made it possible for you to stay in your home for the past four-and-a-half years. And now I am going to bed. I love you," I add, softly touching her hand. I mouth a *thank you* to Jo Ann—who still looks shell-shocked—for being there to help her to bed, and escape toward my bed and my cat.

"I love you too, Gretchen," follows me, "but I make my own decisions." I pause on the steps but don't respond. Is she going to add, *you're not the boss of me?* Her words about my father don't touch me. I knew what she said that day we said goodbye to him was true, but I never understood why, even in grief, she said them. But I know he is not displeased with me now. I have redeemed myself.

When I get to my sanctuary I call Rebecca.

"Mama says she's not moving," I sob, panicked. "She thinks I just want the house and her money, and I'm kicking her out!"

"What! That is ridiculous!"

"And she said Daddy would be unhappy with me." I cry harder.

"Oh for God's sake," she says. "I'm sorry. And that is not true."

When I calm down, she tells me she thinks she knows what happened.

"Stan was at the house today doing yard work and helping Mama with her tapes. Bonnie called me and said she overheard him tell Mama she shouldn't have to move. He told her he would come and live with her, and that he's a good cook."

"What the hell!" I shout. "What a fucking opportunist!"

"I know. That's not going to happen, and we'll deal with it. Try to get some sleep now."

I go to bed, but get no sleep. I'm furious with Stan. I've always considered him a gentle partner in this caregiving adventure, but suddenly he is the opposition. Mama would never be pulled into the wiliness of a telephone scam, but she does not see Stan's offer for what it is: taking advantage of their friendship to secure housing for himself. She had finally accepted the move and now has found her resurrection in him. She's never comprehended what I do behind the scenes. Apparently Stan, who is way out of line in any case, doesn't get that either. I have heard of caregivers scamming their employer, but I never thought Stan would.

∾

We can't drag Mama kicking and screaming out of the house, even figuratively. I'm sick to my stomach. I didn't think this would be so hard.

67

November

Stages of Grief

"I want my bedroom left as it is. If I come back to visit in the summer—if I'm still alive—and walk on the deck, I might want to lie down on my bed to rest."

We have slid into November, and it's Jo Ann's last night. The four of us are having dinner together. Though the move hasn't been mentioned since the night of her outburst two days ago, it's probably always on Mama's mind, as it is on mine.

"Of course," I say, my hopes hardly daring to rise, even as my heart breaks a little bit. *Denial. Anger. Bargaining.* "Nothing will change. And you will be back to visit before summer. We'll bring you up often."

I go to bed, breathing again. Jo Ann is on duty for one more night. I turn off the monitor and sleep a heavy dreamless sleep, waking to a cloudy sky shot with pink-and-orange stripes across the horizon as the rising sun lights up the mountain. Shards of light in the darkness.

The fog is about to roll back in.

❧

While Jo Ann talks to Mama about what furniture and artwork she might like to move to her new home, Rebecca and I go to the Manor to sign the contract and pay the first month's fees. We are hoping to ease Mama into the move before she changes her mind again. The director goes through each page of the contract with us and I ask questions. Rebecca is oddly silent, then begins to cry.

"Do we need to step out for a minute?" I ask. She nods.

Out in the hall, she sobs. "I can't do this! She's going to hate it here! I don't think they can take care of her."

I don't know what to say. I don't know what to do. I wait.

"We're moving too fast. We didn't look at all the options."

"But we did," I protest gently. I've become too accustomed to the roadblocks to be affected anymore. The clouds swallow up the light.

"We didn't look at what full-time care at home would cost." She seems angry now. At me.

"Laurel said upwards of twelve thousand dollars a month," I remind her.

"But we didn't see what it costs in this town. A friend told me it wasn't that much for her mother."

Laurel works in this county, so her estimate is probably accurate. And there are more issues than money. I'm frustrated, but I know it will go badly for everyone if I push it.

"Do we need to wait on this?" I ask. She nods, unable to speak. I'm numb.

∾

We've never been a family that talked about the "tough stuff." In fact, disagreeing was actively discouraged. It's no wonder this emotion-charged conversation and decision is so difficult. I'm stuck between needing to take care of myself and not knowing how to do it without making everyone angry at me.

In the midst of the indecision, I have thought hard about what I want for myself if Mama moves and how I will adjust to the possibility that she stays at home. I'm sad to think of giving up my dream of returning our family property to glory and finding a way to share it. And I'm familiar with giving up what I thought would be—or might be—changing course as necessary. I've been cautiously excited over the prospect of a small place of my own to live, maybe in another town, if it comes to that.

I am clear: my time is up. I know what I need in my life, and where I am willing to compromise to care for Mama and where I am not. Our relationship has become adversarial. I need to heal it if I can before it's too late. I need to be her daughter. Only her daughter. I can't do that and live under the same roof.

There is a departure coming. I just don't know whose or to where.

∾

Several days after Jo Ann returns home to Virginia, Mama is silent about the move, and there has been no conversation among my sisters. Then I learn from Jo Ann that Rebecca has contacted her with concerns and heartache. Jo Ann writes that they are not comfortable with moving forward right now. She has taken a stand after weeks of carefully not taking sides—nor offering input—and it's not with me. I'm back in the far reaches of the fun house mirrors. Alone. I'm not comfortable with lack of consensus either, and I won't jeopardize my relationship with my sisters for what might be seen as my own gain. But I am still going to take care of myself. It's no longer a matter of I "can't" go on the way it's been, but I "won't," the subtle change shifting the power and giving me strength.

I apply for Social Security, wishing I had done it as soon as I was eligible. I could have been socking it away while I didn't have to pay room and board. I gained nothing by waiting. I update my resume and draft a cover letter to explain why there's next to nothing on it for the past four-and-a-half years. I start checking Craigslist for jobs and housing. I write to my sisters, telling them I will stay in the area if possible and share responsibilities equally with Rebecca.

I cry. It has been the hardest four years of my life. I feel betrayed by my sisters. The loss of income and contributions to social security and retirement in the waning years of my working life suddenly feels like the dumbest thing I ever did. And now I'm going to lose my dream, the deferred payoff for these years. It's laughable to think I can be hired at sixty-four for work that means something to me and pays a livable wage. I am terrified to the point of nausea.

◦≈◦

Rebecca comes up for dinner. In spite of her misgivings and sorrow, which she continues to keep from Mama, she helps her over the hurdle. I'm cleaning up the kitchen as Mama picks at her salmon. I hear her ask Rebecca about Stan. I know she's been mystified by his absence, but this is the first time she's mentioned it.

"Has Stan talked to you?" she asks.

"No, he hasn't," Rebecca replies. "Mama, his offer to live with you was inappropriate, and it made our decision-making more difficult. He offered a solution that is not ever going to happen. It has caused contention in the family."

I peek into the dining room. Mama's face is impassive as she continues to move food around on her plate.

"Gretchen has given up a lot to keep you at home for three years more than was her plan. Your questioning of her intentions was really hurtful. She doesn't want your money or your home. She doesn't want you to be unhappy."

I'm stunned she is telling Mama this. Mama's head is bowed. Though she's still holding her fork, her hand is motionless.

"It's becoming harder to keep you safe and requires more care than we can give and still live our own lives. If we hired more care for you at home, Gretchen would still have a lot to do, hiring, training, scheduling caregivers. Being in charge when you are unhappy with them." She stops enumerating the tasks, perhaps also thinking of all she would have to do if I move out.

Mama remains silent as Rebecca hugs her and prepares to go home. I stop her at the door.

"Thank you for what you said," I say. "I love you for it. But does it mean you are ready to sign the contract?"

"I still hate it," she says, "but yes. I'm sure you're right that the rollercoaster is confusing to Mama."

If I am the head—the voice of logic—then Rebecca is the heart of the family. She *is* in my corner, and in Mama's corner, even as she deals with her own grief.

ȣ

Rebecca's words hit home with Mama. Though she doesn't talk about it, I know she feels terrible about her role in the conflict. She calls Stan the next morning and tells him she was wrong to have a conversation with him about where she lives, that it's a family matter, that she does need to move, and it's okay.

We won't hear from Stan again for months, and then after one visit, he'll go away for good. I add to my duties what's left of pre-winter yard work, vacuuming, and trying to help Mama with the taping of her epic story.

Mama is suddenly kinder to me and more appreciative than she has been in the past four years. Though she never apologizes, I accept her kindness as regret.

∾

"I had a crazy dream," Mama tells me when I get her up this morning. "I was helping friends move. I was dusting the floor. I had a huge pile of dust balls. The dust mop I found was completely worn out, but I kept trying to use it."

It's a stunning dream; she has worked so hard to keep functioning at the end of this journey, refusing to give in to her diminishing capacity. I wonder again if not having the house cleaned out has been part of her foot dragging. She's looking for closure to her life here on the hill, and there will be none. She's worn out. The house will go on without her.

Michelle, who has returned for a few hours a week on condition that she not have to do any lifting, helps Mama clean out three sock drawers. It takes all morning, but they end up with a pile of discards. I read that while the ship *Arbella* was anchored off the coast of Yarmouth, England, in 1630—waiting for better weather conditions to begin their crossing to Massachusetts—a small group of Puritans risked the white caps on the Atlantic to row back to town to scrub their linen neckerchiefs one more time before setting out for the ultimate wilderness. Cleaning out her sock drawers, asking for her bedroom to remain unchanged, wistfully asking if someday she can come back to walk on the catwalk is human coping that will get Mama through this walk toward the wilderness of death in which she has lost control of the outcome.

Now I'm in anguish again. Could I do nights if I had no responsibility during the day? The agonizing is my own desperate attempt to keep from feeling like the worst kind of daughter.

While I deal with my guilt and Rebecca with her grief and fears, Mama is in better spirits than I have seen her in a long time. She seems to have made peace with the move, or figured out how to pretend. Now that the commitment is made, she seems relieved and ready to go on.

She is a fierce warrior woman. She does not deal well with small changes, but her long history has proven her amazingly resilient and adaptable to big ones. She has adjusted, however clumsily, to myriad health issues in the last third of her life, including exercising a broken kneecap to stronger than the healthy one, surviving the ruptured appendix, dealing with the madness of tinnitus and hearing loss, coping with failing vision and digestive and bowel issues that began long before old age. She has lived twenty years without her partner. Though she complained ceaselessly, never did she lie down and die because it was too hard.

I have a strong sense that all will be well for her after an adjustment period for each of us. Rebecca is equally sure she won't be okay. Truth probably lies somewhere between.

68

Thanksgiving Week

Stretching the Cord

I feel on the verge of a new life force. If these have been the most difficult years of my life, the past twelve weeks have been the hardest months. I feel the shift coming.

While Rebecca works at her store and grieves—still not at peace with the decision—I help Mama decide what she wants to take with her and make lists. Jo Ann flies back across the country the day before the move, for the second time in a month, to help with the transition.

As we sit at the table the night of Jo Ann's return, chatting while Mama finishes eating, Rebecca suddenly explodes in anger at me, cursing me for something I said in jest to Mama.

"What the hell?" I say, my stomach clenching.

"This is not going to work! She should not be moving!" she shouts.

Mama keeps eating, ignoring the drama. Jo Ann's face is impassive.

"And apparently it's on me," I shout back, not even knowing what I said that set her off.

I go to my room without excusing myself, where I throw myself across my bed, sobbing.

No one checks on me, and I don't go back upstairs. I am so tired of being the bad guy. I get into bed and put my pillow over my head. Do other families have rifts about what to do with parents? Do they survive? Will we?

In the morning, nothing is said by Jo Ann or Mama. I don't hear from Rebecca and don't reach out to her.

∿

The day of the move, the neighbors come with their trailer to move a few pieces of Mama's furniture. I clean the detritus off the dresser, including the camera for the baby monitor, which I take downstairs and drop on my bed. We take everything to her new home and set up her room. Hospice has delivered a hospital bed that we think she will be more comfortable in, and to honor her request to keep her bedroom at home intact. I put a poster on the wall we had made for her hundredth birthday party: Mama in her early twenties, with her sister and a friend, sauntering down a narrow dirt road in their golf whites and sunglasses like Charlie's Angels. I want the staff to see she used to be young. Or maybe it's to remind me.

All that's left is Mama.

I wake her from her nap so we can get her to her new home before dark.

"I'm going today?" she says groggily.

I sigh. "That was the plan. Would you rather wait until morning when we're fresh?"

"Yes," she says.

It does seem like a better idea, and by now I expect the delays.

∿

When I go downstairs for the night, there is the monitor camera on the bed where I dropped it. I pull the plug on the receiver on my bedside table and drop it next to the camera and look at them. I have been listening to Mama breathe and snore and talk in her sleep for almost four-and-a-half years. I have checked the video monitor uncountable times to see if she was awake—or breathing—and if she got back from the bathroom okay. I feel nothing but release.

I gather it all up and dump the pieces in a drawer with other miscellaneous electronics I don't know what to do with—including the original staticky monitor without video, evidence of the many trials and advances over the course of this journey. Jo Ann can listen for her tonight. I have cut the umbilicus; it's time to turn toward the future.

ဆ

The next morning, Rebecca joins us at the Manor for breakfast together in Mama's new home. I leave the house early to take a few more things to her room and make last minute adjustments—wanting it to be perfect—while Jo Ann gets Mama there. I meet them in the dining room where Mama declares breakfast delicious, in spite of the scrambled eggs not meeting the light and fluffy demand I accommodate at home. She's trying to be brave.

We head down the hall to her second floor room, she pushing her walker. After exactly the six weeks the orthopedist said it would take—if it happened at all—her bones have healed, and she is back to her pre-fall abilities.

I feel queasy as Jo Ann opens the door and Mama pushes the walker through the small entry between the bathroom and the double closet in the leg of the T-shaped room. There's a pantry with a microwave at the far end of the closet, and the small table my father made in high school wood shop is across from it. It has accompanied her from home to home for seventy years to the month. I hung a recent photograph of my father's "four fabulous females" above it, along with the blue POLST form with its Do Not Resuscitate instructions for EMTs.

Mama pauses there and we hold our collective breath as she looks around. The new beige carpet emits a chemical smell I hadn't noticed before, and I wait for Mama to say it's irritating her nose, but she doesn't say anything.

Sunlight streaks in through the slanted blinds of the double window overlooking the courtyard garden, visible through a large dogwood tree that will mark the change of seasons. Will there be seasons, plural? She won't be able to see it come into bloom, turn to leaf, become bare again, but I hope it will please her to know it's there. Her new La-Z-Boy electric recliner is in the corner near the window; one of her end tables next to it holds her talking clock, a vase of flowers, a book of Mary Oliver's poetry. Her talking book player from the Library for the Blind sits on her mother's gateleg dining table in the adjacent corner, along with her own tape recorder waiting for her to continue her family history project.

Mama still hasn't moved. I can't see her face as I stand in the doorway behind Rebecca, all of us waiting for her to speak. *She doesn't like it,* I think. I can't bear it if she falls apart or complains about something. I fight the urge to run . . . or to throw up.

Her bedside table is next to the hospital bed in an alcove beyond the dresser that stands on the other side of the window. On the dresser is the framed photo of her and my father she chose to bring. They are young, standing near a lake at the farm in Ann Arbor; perhaps the first time she joined him there to meet his family. He's leaning on a canoe paddle, his other arm stretched behind her holding the other paddle. He's smiling into her eyes; she's boldly smiling back into his, twisting her fingers together at the waistband of her striped skirt. It's a small photograph, but even were it bigger she could see it only by heart.

What can she see? What is she feeling? I'm barely breathing. It has taken so long to get here. I'm wracked with grief, guilt, relief. The emotions tumble inside me, crashing into one another in each one's haste to come out on top.

"I never thought it could be like this," she says finally as her eyes well up. Maybe she is just being gracious and accepting for us, but the crack in her voice sounds like her own relief has won over grief, at least for now. I weep my own long held back tears.

❧

After Mama is settled, I head to Seattle. Since I last saw Adrian two weeks ago, he has learned to sit up without falling over and is rocking on his hands and knees. Elliot has memorized a lengthy book and "reads" it to me, then puts a thirty-five-piece puzzle together by himself. He is signed up for the next level of toddler soccer—the one where parents sit on the sidelines. They are stretching the umbilical cord too.

Rebecca sleeps on a pallet on the floor in Mama's new room the two nights I'm away.

❧

I return from Seattle to a house absent my mother. It feels strangely unfamiliar. Early the next morning, as Jo Ann sleeps, the power goes out. It's dark and chilly and deafeningly quiet. I wrap in blankets and sit in the dark. I have returned to the womb while I contemplate the thinning of the cord that had rejoined me and my mother these past years. I wonder where this freedom will take me. Mama is not the only one who will need time to adjust, but she raised a fierce warrior woman in her image. Though the cord won't be cut through until she leaves the earth, I am ready to meet the future.

69

Year's End

Alone

Four days after the move, we bring Mama back to the house for Thanksgiving dinner. Emma and Wynne, Elliot and Adrian, and my niece and nephew come down from Seattle for dinner. Mama is glad to be with the family, but it tires her. She seems eager to go "home" when it's time.

While the others clean up after dinner, I sit with her out of the commotion where we always sat: she in her favorite recliner she didn't want to take with her because she "never liked it," I at the end of the sofa close to the chair.

"I love thinking of this property as a retreat center," she says out of nowhere.

I freeze, astounded. I hadn't told her my fragile dreaming for the property, so sure she would tell me all the reasons I couldn't do it, but she says it without caveat. How did she know?

"I can imagine it," she adds.

I'm too choked up to speak. "Thank you," I manage to squeak out. "I'm glad you like the idea."

"Your daddy would be pleased too," she says, making amends for her previous outburst. I accept it as apology.

"Thank you for saying that," I say through my tears.

It has mystified me that she hasn't been excited that I want to stay in this home she and my father created and that she has kept going for the past twenty years, a testament to the sense of place she has nurtured. Maybe she doesn't want us to be burdened with an "old house" when she is gone. Saving us from the house and its contents was her last task as a mother, and it wasn't fulfilled.

Later, when I mention the conversation to Jo Ann, she tells me she talked with Mama about my retreat center idea, not realizing I hadn't. She is chagrinned, but I am grateful. It feels like a breakthrough, the edge of a new "sharing" relationship.

⟡

Jo Ann and the rest of the family return to their lives the day after Thanksgiving. On Saturday I wake up alone in the house. I lie in bed marveling. I feel like an enormous weight has been lifted from my shoulders and now I finally can look ahead. It's been raining endlessly, and the valley is flooded, but today the sun is going to come out.

I go upstairs and sit in the corner chair with my mug of steaming coffee and foamy milk to wait for the sunrise. All the shades are up. The sky turns pale pink, then rosy, then streaked with light and color that reflect in the water below. As the sun slides into blinding view, my heart bursts open.

⟡

As November turns to true winter, my optimism vanishes, overcome by the day-to-day reality of Mama's struggle to adjust to her own new life. As her dementia deepens, so does her denial of it. It's hard to help her when we don't know what's real. The myriad things she complains of have all transpired in the past three hours in her mind, though they could have happened days ago, weeks even. Or not at all. I try to stop correcting her memory. I drag up David's words: the invention of fact is not important. I pretty much fail, as I have in the past; it makes me crazy. "It was last week the minister from the church came and stayed too long, not today. Remember?" I say it as if she were simply choosing not to remember. "And according to the log, he only stayed fifteen minutes," as if it mattered how long he stayed if it felt too long.

"You need to have your brain tested, Gretchen," she says, pulling out her go-to defense.

It's her body doing data storage now, and perception is all that matters. I read that virtually none of the memory-impaired believe themselves to be so. My mother inhabits a very large island of comrades, but they each live there alone. She has stepped into a place I cannot go, and it's not my job to drag her back to my world. Harder than trying to pull her back is to give up the attempt.

ᔕ

David tells me it takes at least three months for an elderly person to adjust to a new living situation. It seems optimistic. To adjust to a move while visually impaired at a hundred years old is unfathomable to me. We teach her to leave her room by herself, always turning right out of the door and walking the square of halls clockwise so her room will always come up on the right. We leave a note on the inside of her door, reminding everyone who walks with her to always do the same. She counts the steps and memorizes the locations of the scattered benches—of which she can see the shape—so she knows when it's time to watch for her door. She never makes a mistake, telling everyone her door is the only one with a basket on it—the placement of which was her idea—but she's terrified that she will walk into someone else's room.

My mother's absence in the house is palpable. Maybe it will take me three months to adjust too. I still hear her walker hitting the door jambs, the constantly flushing toilet, her heavy shuffling footfalls, and her soft snore over the phantom monitor. I still glance at her recliner, surprised not to see her slumped over in sleep. The rooms echo with memories of my childhood, and the storage room cabinets bulge with my parents' life before I existed, carefully packed into taped-shut boxes. The past crowds around me, making it difficult to see the future. The house has become my mother, and now it is in control.

∾

We have retained her three private caretakers for two hours a week each so she has company. They read to her, walk the halls with her, clean her room, and occasionally take her out in the car for a haircut or groceries. Bonnie reports she is less "cranky," even sweet. Laurel reports Mama no longer pulls out her parade of physical ailments when she checks in on her. I worry she will be kicked out of hospice again.

If she doesn't complain to others, she shows no such reticence with me. As I listen to her complaints, I tell myself I can hear them, try to give her what she needs, and then go home and light a fire. My life, at least, is better, and I let that be okay, trying to minimize my guilt. As the year ends, her ghost in the house slowly fades and the house seems to open up to me just a bit, to beg a new story even as its walls retain the old one. It sighs with relief and springs toward new life as I clear the clutter and apply fresh paint. But I still don't feel free to fully inhabit the space.

These years have been a reprise of my years as a stay-at-home parent of young children, when moments for my interests—spent with one ear listening for nap to be over—were a footnote to my real life. Now I'm getting ready to make plans further into the distance than I have dared peer for the past four-and-a-half years. Plans in which caring for Mama is now only a piece of the pie. I'm still the daughter on duty, more equally shared now with Rebecca, but it's become more the garden variety caregiving: from afar, lives separate, primary care left to others.

I can't control Mama's days, and I don't need to, because mine are no longer as contingent on hers. I have stepped into new territory too, one she can't control—and for the first time since my return, she has stopped trying to. The two became one, and now we are two again. It feels like a divorce. It feels like giving up. It feels like breaking a vow. It feels like betrayal. It feels like freedom.

∽

I sift through my ideas for the property for a place to begin while Mama lives on. I want to share the property; I need an income; I don't want to have to do a lot of work while so much time is still given to Mama's care; I don't want to overstep my bounds as co-owner of the house. I stayed in an Airbnb when I went to my aunt's memorial service in Tucson, and I wonder if I could do that. It would mean vacating the apartment. Could I move upstairs? Is it time? I start researching.

Mama is searching for what's next too. When she succumbed to the inevitability of the move on the condition that her bedroom at home not be changed, perhaps she harbored some hope she could move back, that this was merely a trial of short duration, in spite of evidence against it. Now, after just over a month, she wants her full-size bed. The hospital bed isn't comfortable and it's too narrow to hold what she needs close by to get through the night: a flashlight in case she needs a beacon in the dark, her talking clock to keep her company, her hearing aid box. She wants her familiar. Maybe it's an admission that she has a new home. Reclaiming my own familiar, I move my bed that's been in storage over the carport into Mama's empty room and purchase a mattress for it. But I don't sleep there. It's not time.

Cautiously, though, I set about making other living spaces more mine. I move my coffee table and an area rug from my basement quarters to the living room, shift my kitchen items to the front of the cabinets and put some of Mama's in a box, and haul out her old Royal manual typewriter from the storage room to decorate a new writing space at my father's desk. I don't discard anything; nothing is mine to make unilateral decisions about.

I'm overwhelmed by the stuff, as Mama must have been. I'm angry with my father, in his refusal to move to a smaller space as my mother wanted, for leaving the accumulation of over half a century of marriage and parenthood for her to dispose of alone. How could any of us have ever thought she could do it by herself? Now I wonder if my intention to stay here myself is to put off relegating the artifacts of a life to the landfill and thrift shops, as if their presence in boxes on shelves can keep my parents and my youth with me.

70

Spring

Death and Life

The past six months have been filled with endings. Mama's sister-in-law died as the leaves turned red and gold, her own sister died in the throes of winter, and my father's last sibling left as grey continued to fold around the Pacific Northwest. Now, as spring contemplates arrival, our neighbor unexpectedly dies. This gentle woman has been my mother's neighbor for more than fifty years, and one of her last remaining close friends. We take Mama to sit by her bed a few days before the end, where she holds Sandy's hand in both of hers and weeps as she seldom has when friends have died in the past years, by degrees leaving her behind.

She has another dream. "I was in the woods looking for a place to sleep. There was a family there too, trying to find a place to lie down and to get away from 'the enemy.' I don't know if the enemy was loggers or what. I woke up and had to shake my head and figure out where I was. It wasn't a bad dream, just complicated and surreal." She is the last one standing of her generation in our long-lived family. I can't imagine what that feels like, but maybe her dream, and that it didn't frighten her, holds a clue.

There have been beginnings too. I talked to my sisters about opening an Airbnb, and they gave their blessing. I moved upstairs to Mama's bedroom. I patched the cat-scratched love seat I brought from North Carolina for my downstairs living area and hired someone to replace the bathroom floor and do minor repairs. I took photos and designed my pages on the Airbnb website and gave my corner of paradise a name: Three of Earth Farm. In the tarot, the threes represent resolution of the one and two. This property began with its purchase in 1960 (the ace), it was tested when my father died in 1995 and in my mother's will to keep it up (the two), and now we three sisters are accepting the mantle (the three). Three of Earth, in my Gaian Tarot deck, represents gathering in community to create something of lasting value: a place of abundance, harmony, and pleasure.

I go live online and wait for my first reservation.

☙

It's been the wettest winter and early spring in Pacific Northwest recorded history. I've been taking my Vitamin D, which my doctor says everyone who lives in the PNW should take. I don't get depressed by the lack of the natural source, but I'm getting a little grumbly. Then spring creeps in on a foggy mid-April morning.

I sit in the quiet cocoon of fog, anticipating the beautiful morning that almost always follows fog. I watch four deer through the window, grazing under the apple trees below the house, appearing and disappearing in the mist. I sip my coffee in the blanket of silence as I go through my seed packets to find the April planters—March planters in a warmer year.

When the sun begins to glow behind the veil, I dress quickly in the cold house and go outside. I gather my tools in the wheelbarrow and head to the garden. The air is invigorating, but not as uncomfortable as I expected. I round the curve in the driveway. The sky is already brilliant blue over the meadow, the sun casting shadows across the sparkling dew-damp grass. The birds are singing, the mourning doves are looking for a mate, an owl is hooting its way off to sleep, a sapsucker taps its way to breakfast at the top of a utility pole. I stop in my tracks, overcome. Two months too long of rain and grey, and all is forgiven.

I watch a honking skein of geese fly overhead, and my heart soars with them; I feel a stirring. My mother's love of mountains and trees and flowers and this earth is the life blood that runs through my veins. It is the beauty that gave her a rich and splendid life. I'm sad that after all the years of breathing the damp earth, the flowers, the cleansing rain, Mama's nostrils are filled now with the odors of residents' cats, adult diapers, institutional food, and ammonia. I will take her some fresh rosemary for her vase.

∽

As the reluctant spring continues to seep in through cracks and crevices, Mama seems to be coming out of her annual winter slump. She shows signs of adjusting to her new home. She stages a sit-in at lunch, refusing to leave the dining room or have her plate removed until the director comes upstairs so she can tell her about the lack of crab in the crab cakes. She joins the resident council after that and meets with others to air their grievances to the staff, mostly about the food. The "inmates" as she calls them—mostly women who are, no doubt, not cooking for themselves and others for the first time since they left their mother's kitchens—bond around their food complaints. Her work in the world as an advocate and a rebel continues.

I try to keep the strong woman she has been over the past century in my heart when I get exasperated with her. I want her to know before she leaves that I saw all she was; I want her to forget my impatience with her. In my humanness, I know I can't completely eliminate my irritation, but for both our sakes, in the time we have left together, I do my best to swallow it in favor of kindness. And forgive myself when I fail.

I get better at listening to her complaints without engaging. I stop telling her she has a bad attitude. I stop trying to get her to tell me something good that happened. Having an opinion reminds her of her own humanity, especially with her short-term memory in free-fall. I change the subject when there's a break in the action and tell her what's happening on the hill and in my life, and then I get to go home. Some days I can keep the light lit inside me.

And once again she is too healthy for Medicare to authorize hospice's services, and Mama loses Laurel's weekly reassurances. We all lose the peace of mind that comes with knowing the team will be there to help us navigate the next bowel blockage.

◠

"You're a hundred-year-old miracle," I told Mama the other day. She had been to the house for brunch with Emma, Wynne, and the boys. She marveled that her incontinence briefs were dry when I finally helped her to the toilet before taking her home. She is rarely and barely incontinent. "What I'm worried about, Gretchen, is my heart," she said in response.

A few days later, I decide to get to the bottom of her fears, if there is a bottom. "How is the pain around your heart?" I ask, missing Laurel's assurance that it's gas.

"It's gone away," she says.

"When you have those pains, you are eager to have your blood pressure taken and to have a doctor tell you what's going on. Can you tell me what you want them to do? What are you afraid of?"

"I'm afraid of being in pain for a long time. I don't want medication. I want to die quickly."

"I think if it's a heart attack you will go quickly, as you hope. But more likely your heart will stop beating someday, probably while you are sleeping, but that isn't the same as a heart attack. I don't think it will hurt."

"Okay," she says quietly.

She is—we are—in the anteroom now, and we might be here for a long time. It's a dark and mysterious place; frightening to her, curious to me.

I change the subject, deciding to tell her about my Airbnb, which has welcomed its first two guests. It's risky, but if to change our relationship is why I came, I have to keep trying. I fill my voice with enthusiasm and my words with excitement, hoping to clue her in to the response I'm hoping for.

"You are going to let strangers sleep in the house?"

I let my disappointment go with a sigh. "I put locks on the interior doors so guests can't get into the rest of the house. I'm excited to meet new people and share what you and Daddy so lovingly created. Last week's guest was a photographer. He took an early morning walk in the natural area. He said it was beautiful, and asked me to thank you for saving the trees. Connections are how we change the world, one stranger at a time. It's what you did. It's what I can do."

She brightens at my words but doesn't say anything more.

71

Summer

Milestones

We began birthday month with another forty-hour tour of duty in the hospital. Thanks to the vigilance of Bonnie, Mama's private caregiver who also works at the Manor, we caught the bowel obstruction—the third one in ten months—in its early stage.

The obstruction cleared quickly and forty-eight hours after discharge we celebrated Mama's 101st birthday at the Manor with family from Seattle, a few old friends, and several fellow residents. It pleased me to walk around the circle in the dining room serving a bite-sized cupcake from our favorite caterer, a single fresh strawberry, and a tiny cup of pink lemonade to the residents I have come to know in the sevenfold amen of their lives. It felt like communion.

And the best gift—compliments of the blockage—hospice is back.

❧

I celebrate my sixty-fifth birthday, the summer solstice, and the fifth anniversary of my return home by getting the claustrophobic branches of the Douglas fir tree trimmed up as I promised myself I would do when Mama was no longer here, though I thought she would be farther gone than across town. I have heard the geese honking through the valley, but couldn't see them. I've watched the hawks making lazy circles in the sky, but only at the end of the valley, losing them behind the tree when they came close. I couldn't see the rising sun's glow over the mountain from my corner chair in the living room. It's a symbolic "reawakening."

When the first huge branch is gently lowered to the ground, the open sky slams against my chest, throwing it open. I weep as more branches come down. I cry for my father so long gone from this panorama he loved, and for my mother, here so long but unable to see the rainbows through her nearly sightless eyes. Eight enormous boughs. I barely need to breathe any more, the air coming from so deep through my expanded chest. I thank the branches for their beauty, the shade they provided for my mother's damaged ancient eyes, their shelter for the birds and squirrels. I welcome the sky.

∾

My time with Elliot and Adrian every week is almost over, two school years with a year off between. School ends soon, and Wynne will be home for the summer; Adrian will join Elliot in day care in September.

Mama walked independently when I arrived. Five years later she is unsteady, even supported by full-time walker use, gripping it like a lifeline with one hand as she stretches her other arm out for something else to grab when she sits down. One-year-old Adrian is at the exact crossing point with her: about to take his first wobbly independent steps, but for now continuing to hold on to anything he can reach. His legs will become stronger and then his confidence will be unstoppable. He will fall and get up, fall and get up. Before we know it he will be running full tilt. The day will come when Mama won't get up from her chair without assistance, as her weakening legs threaten to collapse. She will graduate to a wheelchair. One day she will not get up at all. The timetable is less certain than Adrian's, but it will surely come to pass if she lives long enough.

Three-year-old Elliot has rocketed beyond his great-grandmother, learning new words as fast as she forgets the large vocabulary she has commanded for decades. He recites the simple text of library books after hearing them one time; she can't hang onto what she was just told, though she recalls the poems she memorized in school. Reciting them in her head brings her comfort when she can't sleep at night.

These tender years with Elliot and Adrian are a gift that will forever be the melody weaving through the thrumming bass of these discordant years. Although their brains will forget the year I spent with each of them, I hope a knowledge that they were well loved by their Gigi as they began exploring their world will remain in some hidden space within them. As my mother comes to the end of her exploring, I hope in some hidden space she feels well loved too.

year six

72

Autumn

Connections

I took an epic number of hikes over the summer, taking full advantage of my freedom with Mama receiving care I don't have to provide or find for her. If I remember these days when I'm an old-old, I want to be able to say to everyone, "I had fun getting old."

But I want more than to remember. I want it to be who I am—my essence—when I am no longer able to hike the hike, drive the drive, drink the nectar. I want my children to refuse to listen to my complaints about bowel function, the terrible food, how forgetful other people are, and to ask me instead about what I did with my one beautiful life. I hope the wanting will make it so.

My mother was a hiker too, especially as a young woman in the Great Smoky Mountains National Park. I use my outings as connection; it is the best one we have. Sometimes it works.

After a long hike in July to Indian Henry's Hunting Ground, a meadow in Mt. Rainier National Park that was home to a Native American guide who lived and hunted there before it became a park, I sat on the stool at Mama's knee to tell her about it.

"I was there many years ago," she told me.

"It was a steep climb!" I said. "I was exhausted."

"I remember. And did you cross a river?"

"Yes," I said.

"Was there a cabin in the meadow?"

"Yes. And the wildflowers were knee high as I walked through the meadow on the footpath!"

"And could you see the mountain at the edge of the meadow?"

"It was a beautiful day. The mountain was out full on."

"Oh, my dear daughter," she whispered. "I'm so glad you got to see it."

∼

My efforts to distract Mama from her complaints by asking her to tell me stories is seldom successful. The immediacy of each day thieves her attention. She is constipated again this week, and sure she has a blockage in spite of the on-call hospice nurse hearing bowel tones and the lack of other blockage symptoms. Laurel is on vacation, and Mama doesn't trust the substitute. I spend my days with her, heating soup, bringing special-order food from the dining room, reading to her, silently listening to her complaints. She doesn't get dressed for days.

On the fourth day, with Rebecca on early duty, I try to wash off fatigue in the shower after a night of not sleeping because Smudge, who is eighty-four in cat years, is constipated and pooping outside the litter box again. She meowed all night. Soon I will have to make an end-of-life decision for her. She alternately sits on the bathmat and on the edge of the tub meowing. I lose it, slapping my hands on the tile wall over and over, crying and screaming at her to go away and stop *whap* fucking *whap* whining *whap, whap, whap*! "Meroow, meroow, meroow," she says from the mat as I sob. I don't want this to be my life anymore. I want to be fully free.

⁓

When I arrive in Mama's room late morning she tells me she had been waiting for the aide who said she was going to make her some cereal. I ask the aide when I see her. She says they had not had that conversation.

I make her Malt-o-Meal, and we walk three rounds of the hall. A dozen residents and staff stop us to ask Mama how she is feeling and tell her they miss her in the dining room. They are a family looking out for their own, and she has come to accept them as such. "I'm much better," she tells them all, cheerfully.

Back in her room, she rejects my suggestion that she sit up in her recliner for a while, wanting to get back in bed. She was fine in the hall, but I brace myself for the next round of complaints. As usual, I can't get the bedding right or the rice bags correctly positioned.

When she is finally settled, I give her a kiss and start to edge toward the door.

"Rebecca will be here after work," I say. "I'll see you in the morning."

"Do you have any R & B guests?" she asks, one of her acronyms for my Airbnb, along with R & R and B & R.

"I do," I say, reluctantly sitting back down in the chair by her bed to tell her their story.

She nods. *Is that approval?*

"Thank you for reading me your blog about your hike at Paradise," she adds. "Don't forget to read me the rest of the chapters about your camping trip to Mt. Hood."

What is happening here?

"Have you started your writing group yet?"

"Did you make scones or muffins this week at the deli?"

I didn't even know she was listening when I told her my plan to facilitate a writing circle of women, and about my newest little job.

"What are you going to do when you get home?"

"Take a nap," I say.

It's the closest to a conversation about my life we've ever had.

"Thank you, dear Gretchen," she says as I say goodbye again. "I'm proud of you. You are so . . ." she struggles to find the right word, ". . . interesting," she finishes.

It is the best tribute she could have paid me. And the most stunning—it's not a word I've ever thought of to describe myself. I return to the car and sit with my head on the steering wheel and sob.

This is why I needed to come home. And now she's leaving me.

73

Winter

Letting Go

I return from a too short trip to North Carolina to see Max and Ethan and their parents, afraid to be away long. It's just the third time I have traveled across the country to spend time with these sweet, swiftly growing grandsons, and they have been here only twice. It's a choice I knew I was making when I moved, and it continues to break my heart.

Mama is glad to see me. I tell her about my trip and the boys—her older great-grandsons. When I kiss her goodbye and head for the door, she stops me with an out-of-the-blue question: "How is Smudge?"

I turn back, surprised; she's never asked about my cat. "I guess she's okay. Sort of. She's old." I don't know what to say.

"She's had a long life and given you joy. You've been through a lot together."

My eyes fill up. "We have traveled a long distance together. Thank you for asking about her." I come clean then, she's given me a rare opening to share emotions. "I've been struggling over letting her go. I don't think she is suffering, but I can't know for sure. She isn't enjoying life much though. And I'm not enjoying her much."

I begin to forget who we're talking about.

"You will miss her, and grieve her absence," she says gently, "but maybe it's time to let her go."

Mama might know exactly who she is talking about.

"I will miss her." My eyes fill again. I give Mama a closer hug and another kiss before I leave.

❧

Smudge doesn't eat, drink, or walk if she doesn't want to; she sleeps because she can. I look into her eyes, and those mountain-lake-deep pools of green are blank clouds. Like Mama's faded blue eyes, the light has gone out.

I can choose to release her from this existence that is barely existing, and I'm getting ready, knowing I am opening myself to the vulnerable place of choosing grief before grief chooses me. I tell her it's okay to let go. She has never been a snuggly cat, but now she relaxes into my arms and looks back at me and I recognize that she is telling me it's okay to let her go.

Mama is ready to leave too, and there's not a damn thing I can do to help her out of here. Everyone says, "Your mother is doing great! How wonderful!" No, she is not doing great. She can walk, pushing her walker in endless loops around the hall. She can feed herself, but mostly with her fingers now—unable to see to connect utensil with bite—and it embarrasses her. She only occasionally enjoys what she eats. She walks because she has to, she eats because she has to, she drinks fluids because she has to; she refuses to enjoy napping, and yet napping is all she can do.

I get ready to say goodbye to Smudge. I'm almost out of insulin and don't want to buy another $180 vial. Then she has a sugar crash: too much insulin. I put corn syrup on her gums and hold her until her legs can support her again. I reduce the dosage. Of course that stretches the bit of insulin in the bottom of the vial, buying me time to change my mind, for her to give me a clearer sign one way or another.

⌒

Two weeks later I'm still agonizingly looking for clarity. "Give me a sign. Please," I beg Smudge. I've responded to her wailing, loss of appetite, weight loss, excess shedding, dehydration, and lethargy by adjusting her insulin. *What the hell kind of sign do you want?* she seems to ask.

I want concrete evidence, that's what I want; something I can't fix with an injection a couple times a day. I don't want to feel like I killed her because I was tired of interrupted nights and cleaning up vomit. But I don't get to choose the easy way out. She needs me to be in charge because she can't be.

From my perspective, this has been a better week than she's had in a long time. She didn't throw up or walk wonky. Though she is still constipated from dehydration, she keeps it in the litter box. She joins me in the living room to sleep on my lap in the evenings and entreats me for scratch time in bed again. *She's better! She's telling me she wants to stay.*

But I've heard that humans at life's end seem to rally before they slip into death. Is that what this is? Or is she saying she's *not* ready? When Mama asks about my life, is she needing to make sure I know I am loved before she leaves? Or has her will to live made a comeback? I have to make the appointment to help Smudge go soon or keep propping her up as she yo-yos her way to the inevitable last breath.

In the late day setting sun, the appointment with the vet still not made, I notice the maple tree at the corner of the house. Yesterday it was brilliant red, today all the leaves are on the ground, blanketing the spot where Smudge will be buried.

She starts her mournful crying again in the middle of the night, begging for a drip in the bathtub and continuing to cry after I turn it on. It isn't enough to satisfy her thirst, but she won't drink from her bowl. She is restless, on and off the bed using the stool she needs to make the leap. Neither of us sleep as my monkey mind turns over and over.

The owl hoots, closer than usual, a single haunting call through the fog beyond the open window. Smudge lies down on my legs, finally still. My mind quiets then, and I fall into a brief sleep and dream of her stalking shrews in the phlox at the back of my yard in North Carolina.

∽

When the vet's office opens, I call and make an appointment for Friday morning when Rebecca can go with me. And then I sob. I weep in relief for the decision, in grief for the loss, in gratitude for seventeen years with this companion, longer than any cat I've had—and only a year short of the longest live-in human relationship I've had.

I decorate a box to put her now thin body in and dig a hole under the bare maple before the rains come.

∽

I bury Smudge under the maple, where life will go on above her. Each spring buds will burst with new life; in summer green leaves will be the playground for birds and squirrels; autumn will bring dazzling crimson, a last hurrah before rain and snow batter and bend the bare branches through the long winter sleep. And then spring will return in the endless cycle.

I sit in the rain next to her on the stump of the old big leaf maple, the tree my father climbed on a sunny day in 1958 and saw Mt. St. Helens, deciding this was the land on which he and my mother would build their home. I see him caring for the grounds and my mother the house. I hear their voices and feel their love. My father left too soon. My mother stayed too long. I don't know if I will feel the loss of her as deeply as I do my father. I don't know if I will be able to grieve at all, the relief so great.

But I already miss Smudge and her little black-and-white face that accompanied me through the loss of a relationship and a trip across the country, and who snuggled up next to me when I finally fell into bed each night of these challenging years. Could it be that I will miss my mother too? I can't imagine it. Tears become one with the rain.

74

Year's End, 2017

Mother Lode

A month ago, at the one-year anniversary of her move to the Manor, Mama told Laurel that a year ago was hard. She hadn't wanted to leave her home, she wished she had died instead. "But now," she told her, "it's okay. It was the right thing to do, and I'm glad to be where I am."

Rebecca and I are moving on with our lives as Mama clings by her fingernails to hers. I'm coming to the end of the first series of the women's writing circle I'm facilitating, maintaining the family property, visiting my Seattle family, running a successful Airbnb, occasionally baking at the deli, managing Rebecca's online store, and hiking solo on high mountain trails in this beautiful corner of the country. I resigned the remote job I've had for four-and-a-half years that wasn't bringing me joy. Rebecca was elected to the city council and is running her business from an alternate storefront while dealing with insurance and yet-to-begin repairs on her building that was crashed into by a drunk driver six months ago. Our lives are full even as we remain dutiful in the care of our mother.

In spite of her gloom, in her own resilient way, Mama has adjusted to her new home. I walk the halls with her, read her newspaper articles about her locally world-famous daughter, argue with her about one thing and resist argument about something else, set her straight on one egregiously fabricated story while ignoring most. When she tells me I need to get my memory checked after I tell her she didn't ask me to take her favorite sweater to the cleaners, I just say I will take it, though her false accusations of me and others remain one of the hardest things to let be. I tell her stories about her four great-grandsons, and she says not seeing who they become is her only regret about leaving. I heat her rice bags for her increasingly frequent naps while half listening to her complaints about the staff. I adjust her bedding and put artificial tears in her eyes.

Then the rays of the sweet person she is at her core sneak around her discontent like the sun on an overcast day, as if she suddenly remembers who she is: "I still enjoy being alive in this world. Thank you for being here with me, my sweet daughter. I love you so much."

My heart warms, and I remember who she is too. It is a sliver of light in the vast cloud-filled sky. However annoyed we are with each other, however demanding she is and resentful I am, as I leave her after a visit now, she never fails to tell me what seemed to slip her mind these years since I came back home: "I love you. Thank you for all you do. Thank you for being here."

I moved across the country and into my mother's home at the beginning of my seventh decade looking for the relationship I'd never had with my mother. I wanted her to accept and love me for who I was, not for who she expected me to be. I longed for a mother who was my best friend, my support staff, but what I got was advice and skepticism. Perhaps if she knew me, I thought, things would be different.

But maybe a cheerleader was never what I needed. Maybe I have needed to hike solo all along. I let my husband and later my partner be my backbone and then rejected them because I could never locate my Self there after abdicating it to them. But my mother has been setting a quiet example ever since my father died, showing me how to be my own champion. As I read the letters my parents wrote to each other in their twenties, and see her image in grainy old photographs, imagining her beyond the white borders, I see a fierceness that has always resided at her core. Perhaps inadvertently, she has been teaching me to recognize who I am and what I can do, to find what dreams motivate me and to follow the path. And she has shown me that it's never too late.

Several times I heard her say that her eighties were her favorite decade. She had just turned seventy-nine when my father died; her declaration confounded me. "What made it your favorite?" I finally ask.

"I was independent," she says. "Though it was sometimes overwhelming, I discovered I was capable of making decisions. During my marriage," she goes on, warming to the topic, "I felt like George was in charge of everything, and he didn't include me in decision-making."

It rocks me to hear that she had squashed her soul as I had. Neither of us knew how to be strong in a relationship and let the other person be strong alongside us. Her activism after her children left home was the beginning of a tsunami of independence, but my father's death set her free to fully claim her power. It's no wonder she never asked her daughters for help making decisions—it was her time. Surely these years spent under the same roof felt like control was being wrested from her again, as it did for me. It was the trying to hold onto our Selves—as perhaps we were fifty years ago—that put us at loggerheads, each other the only foe we fought for it.

When she thanks me for being here with her and tells me she loves me, sometimes saying that I'm amazing, I squint my eyes and can imagine pompoms waving for me in her time-worn hands. I will never find my completion from her—it's not hers to give. If I ever felt my mother tried to crush my courage and initiative, it is my grown-child job to move on and claim my power for myself.

These past five-and-a-half years I have peered into my mother's past trying to figure out how she got to be who she is, that mix of low self-esteem and determined control, hypochondria and over-the-top self-care. But what I needed to know all along is who my mother is now, not how she got here. She is an invincible woman who probably longed for a cheerleader herself and became her own. And she isn't going to let anyone take the pompoms from her hands until her fingers relax into death.

∼

There is more to letting go of a parent at life's end than physical release. As I increasingly believe in my own ability and stand in my own vision of myself instead of waffling with every unsolicited piece of advice, I can wholeheartedly accept her and love her as the mother I got. If she has been disappointed in me, she too is letting it go and embracing the daughter she got. We have, without words, forgiven each other for who we are, in all our imperfections. I hope she has also forgiven herself. I hope I can forgive myself.

As I camp and hike alone, I have gained confidence in my capacity to overcome my fears and trust my strong body. I silence the voice of the mother I heard in childhood and again these past years, telling me I'm not smart enough, strong enough, the right gender to do what I believe I can do. I know she would be appalled that I have felt like she was saying any of those words to me, perhaps believing her undeniable love was enough for me to know she was in my corner, and she didn't need to say so.

My times of solitude provide spaces to shut out the racket and hear my own voice, to recognize my strength, to listen to my soul stirrings and move forward with courage. My mother, who never gave up fighting for herself, has unwittingly taught me one last thing.

I came across the country to show my mother I am capable. I ended up proving my capability to myself. I didn't lose my mind. I found it. I didn't become my mother. I became myself.

Going Home

My mother died while she slept on April 21, 2018—Earth Day weekend—as the dogwood beneath her window at the assisted living facility was budding and the trillium in her beloved woods on the hill were turning pink and purple in their own seasonal death throes. She could see neither, but I told her, and she understood as she still understood nearly everything at fifty-three days short of 102 years.

She had not been feeling well for a few days and, as usual, she had plenty of theories: too many of the refried black beans I finally made for her, first one then another batch; too much 7-Up; too much bacon; food gone bad in the Manor kitchen; unripe tomatoes. And too much of the only food that gave her pleasure, chocolate ice cream, which she requested and received every day.

The on-call hospice nurses had theories too: pneumonia, the flu, a stomach virus. Laurel, though, thought it was what it always had been: a partial bowel blockage. We never finished the conversation with Mama about whether or not to go to the hospital when it happened again, to lie in the cold ER on the skinny, hard gurney and have the nasogastric tube inserted. But she had said several times—and especially the last week—she was ready to die. And so my sisters and

I chose for her. We weren't going. Maybe it was the refried beans that caused the blockage that led to the end. But she enjoyed them, and loved me lavishly for making them for her. That was all that mattered.

"Who knew dying would be so hard," she told Laurel, as we all tried to keep her comfortable, increasing the morphine frequency and then the dosage after thirty-six hours with little sleep. She didn't mean emotionally hard, but that it would be so hard to come by. Perhaps she knew this was the end. She slept through the morning, then, and into the afternoon while I sat in the recliner pretending to read.

We called Jo Ann and the three Seattle grandchildren to come. They would all arrive the next day. Several friends visited as she slept. I called Stan the Handy Man from whom we had been estranged for a year and a half. He came and stayed for a long time, making peace with me and I with him, holding Mama's hand, crying. Somehow we knew it was time to say goodbye, and yet we thought we had time. Maybe we couldn't believe we were going to outlive her.

It seemed she wasn't going to wake up again, but she did. Rebecca and I had several good hours with her. We told her the family was coming. "Good," she said faintly. We told her her friends had been there. We told her about Stan: that he was studying botany at the community college and had told the scholarship board she had been his inspiration. "He must have said Robert," she said, using her depleted energy in typical self-effacement, insisting it was our neighbor, not her, he had honored.

I played the ukulele she had given me for my birthday two years earlier, that I was finally learning to play, stumbling through a familiar bit of "Appalachian Spring." I read Mary Oliver poems to her. I told her what was happening at her beloved home on the hill. That when I'd gone home late the night before there was a yellow-eyed opossum in the driveway.

The hospice team stopped by. They had known her for nearly three years as she went off their service with each surge in vitality and back on with each bowel blockage. She told the social worker to be sure to close the front door so the opossum didn't get in the house—giving instructions on taking care of things at her home when she could barely speak.

She stopped asking for food, except to whisper she had ordered two egg rolls while Rebecca, a dear friend, and I ate take-out Thai in her room. Though her mouth was dry, she didn't ask for water and didn't seem to want the swab I offered. She stopped complaining of being cold, of stomach distress. She let me massage lotion into her hands and feet without shrieking in pain. In retrospect, there were clear signs she was doing what we had been wishing she would do for months, letting go, though we never really knew what that meant nor how she could achieve it. I read that those who stop eating and drinking slowly become euphoric, falling into a peaceful coma. Or maybe it was the morphine. But those last two days, she seemed to be ready and choosing.

She named people to whom we were to express her love. We told her to tell Daddy we loved him. She told us he loved us so much. We said, "We know." She told us she loved us. We said, "We know." We told her we loved her. She said she was proud of us, and thanked us for our generosity of time to her. We told her it was a privilege. We thanked her for being a wonderful mother and told her we were going to be fine. We said and did all that needed to be said and done when you are saying goodbye to the one who gave you life. We felt complete.

Rebecca went home late to bed, because we thought we had time. Jo Ann, arriving in town late, went to the house from the airport to sleep before coming to see Mama in the morning. I tried to rest in the recliner when Mama went back to sleep, on three medications every four hours now: morphine for pain, Compazine that kept at bay the earlier nausea and anxiety, atropine to dry up the secretions that were causing the breath in her chest to rattle.

I couldn't sleep. I held her hand, whispered that I loved her, stroked her thin white hair as she slept.

Please forgive me. I forgive you. I forgive myself. I love you.

When the rattle returned, I sat in the chair next to her bed after pushing her call button at ten minutes till midnight to make sure the med tech brought her three comfort medications on time, my head bowed on the bed next to her, my hand wrapped around hers. "I'm right here, Mommy, I'm right here." Maybe she knew, maybe not. But I knew.

Her hands were cool and clammy, but for the first time ever before the temperature rose in July, she didn't ask for her heated rice bags. She hadn't asked for much of anything that day, except to indicate yes or no to our questions. No to more covers. Yes to the leg and foot massages I offered that I couldn't get anywhere near right twenty-four hours earlier, but then were accepted however I gave them.

All her routines were gone. No frequent requests for drops in her eyes. No bathroom requests. No requests for water. No complaints.

Her breathing was erratic, the Cheyne-Stokes pattern of crescendo and decrescendo that often accompanies heart failure. I listened to her take a shallow breath followed by a long pause and each time wondered if that was the last one. Her living these past years had been that same pattern of brief energy followed by despair followed by another burst.

I sat in the recliner with my computer after that last dose of meds at midnight—she not waking up when they were put under her tongue—documenting what was happening, what I was feeling.

Mama is sleeping with the rattle in her chest that hospice says sounds worse to us than it feels to her. I'm on high alert every time she stops making the sound I wish she would stop making because I want her to be comfortable. Because I'm afraid it will wake her up. Because it sounds frighteningly like the end and suddenly I'm not ready. Because I'm afraid she is taking her last breath and I will miss it. Because I'm afraid I'm too far away. Because I'm afraid.

As I wrote, I heard the rattle stop, vaguely wondering if she was still breathing, subconsciously choosing to finish the paragraph I was typing before I got up to check on her.

Knowing and not knowing she had silently left.

I went to her side then. She was so still. "Mommy," I said softly. "Mommy!" I called a little louder, pushing gently on her shoulder as I had when I was a child waking from a nightmare. No return to shuddered breath. No flutter of anything. Her brow was unfurled, soft, unworried. "Mommy!" I sobbed. "No, Mommy, no!" I howled into her shoulder, kissed her face, keened some more.

I called my sisters just after one in the morning, then crawled to the far side of the double bed she had slept in for five decades— Daddy's side—and gathered her into my arms. It no longer mattered that I might be hurting her fragile body. I rocked her and sang the lullaby she once sang to me, my voice cracking with tears: *Lullaby and good night, with roses bedight . . . lay down now and rest, may your slumber be blessed.*

I was sorry the family was not in time, but perhaps she just needed to know we would be together and she didn't need to see and be seen. She knew she was loved, and that we knew we were loved. It was what she most wanted at the end, and we had said it to each

other every day for weeks. Her work was done, and she slipped away—
without any of the pain she so feared, other than that of lingering too
long—passing the mantle to us without further instruction.

○‿◡

To be with my mother for this passage was a gift I had prayed to
be granted from the beginning of this journey of accompaniment—
this gap "year." Two thousand, four hundred, forty-four days. I had
waited for this for so long, for both of us to be released, and now there
was a hole in the world I felt instantly. One moment it was a place
in which I had a parent, and the next it was not. And my nagging
questions were answered:

Will the relief when it's over be so great that I can't grieve?

*Will I ever be able to hold her essence in my memory untainted by
how hard these years have been?*

How long will it take to let go of the toll exacted?

As I held the empty shell of my mother in my arms and whispered *I love you* in her ear, I already knew.

Gratitudes

I had a village of support during the nearly six years I cared for my mother and wrote down the story. There's no way I can thank all those who were there for me, but here's a beginning.

Thank you to Trader Joe's for cheap wine and dark chocolate, to the Washington Trails Association for the best places to hike, to America the Beautiful Lifetime Senior Pass for half-price camping and free entry to Paradise, and to friends who loaned me their homes so I could escape my life.

To those who read my blog, *Daughter on Duty*: knowing you were out there standing with me, telling your own stories, and thanking me for letting you know you were not alone in your own caregiving, literally saved me from going over the edge.

To Elizabeth Hudson Willingham: I could text anything to you and know you would understand and not judge. And being your shoulder to lean on, when both of yours were weighed down with your own parental caregiving, strengthened me for another day—or at least another hour. And to Vickie Leigh for always being a text away to remind me this was not my forever.

To the Women's Writing Circle for your encouragement of me as a writer and as a teacher, and for continuing to come back to tell your stories.

To Hedgebrook: Women Authoring Change, for a life-giving week of solitude, learning, and food prepared by someone else. And to master teacher, Theo Nestor (*Writing is My Drink*), for her course on memoir structure.

To all my writing teachers, especially Christina Baldwin (The Self as the Source of the Story writing workshop): your mentorship, friendship, encouragement, support, and generosity kept me on the road of writing this story, convincing me *Mother Lode* was a story that needed to be told—and that I could tell it. To all the women of SAS retreats through the five week-long sessions I attended: thank you for sharing your beautiful stories and listening with such encouragement to mine. You are my people. Special gratitude to Joanna Powell Colbert (author/artist of *The Gaian Tarot*) and Janis Hall for our enduring friendship forged at the first SAS gathering in 2012; and—along with Christina—for reading and critiquing via Zoom, every word of my manuscript during the Great Pandemic, and for honoring me with the reading of your works in progress. Long live the Queens.

To Dianne Kozdrey Bunnell Raymond (*The Protest*), Tammy Coia (The Memoir Coach), and Michal Nortness for reading or listening to early terrible drafts of this story. To beta readers Gail Chesson (*I Went Walking*), Cheryl Davenport, Becky Dougherty, Lynn Fena, Bridget Flood (*Blue Hole Wisdom*), Lynn Jarrard, and Pamela Sampel (www.PamelaSampel.com) for offering wisdom that made the story a better read. To the many other people who read or listened to parts of the story.

To Barbara Kenady Fish, my childhood neighbor, horseback-riding buddy, and forever friend, for proofreading the advance reader copy. How poetic that our nature-loving mothers died within two hours of each other on Earth Day weekend.

To Peggy Haymes for permission to use her words for the epigraph: they are a perfect description for this unmapped journey.

To Brooke Warner, Krissa Lagos, Jennifer Caven, Shannon Green, Cait Levin, and the rest of the team at She Writes Press for improving my manuscript and for publishing it.

Deepest gratitude to Michelle, "Stan," Bonnie, Kim, Jill, and Jill, and to the staff at Cooks Hill Manor for providing loving care to my mother, especially when she needed a break from me; to Laurel Fisher and the rest of the hospice team, for your love, patience, care, and support, and for keeping us in hospice service as much as you possibly could; and to David Robinson, for helping me understand how it was for my mother, and for telling me I was vital to her living when I felt like I was failing her.

Though you didn't choose it, thank you, Nicholas, for being your Nana's first caregiver, providing support and presence on the day her partner of 51 years died. She, and all of us, were so grateful you were there.

Deep gratitude to Emma and Wynne for loving your Nana and for trusting me to care for your boys, giving me regular escapes from elder care and time with the younger generations.

To Jo Ann, thank you for your willingness to fly across the country and provide respite care so I could get away. Those were the best weeks.

Most especially, thank you to Rebecca for being in the rabbit hole, the hospital room, and the kitchen with me. You did this by yourself for years, I could not have done it for a week without you.

Finally, forever gratitude to my parents, George and Stellajoe, for creating a home in this amazing corner of the country and filling it with so much love that we all wanted to come back. Kudos for leaving everything in it for us to deal with so we would remember you when you were gone—and so we would know you better in death than we did in life.

About the Author

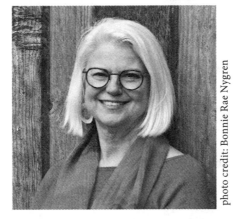

photo credit: Bonnie Rae Nygren

Gretchen Staebler is a daughter, sister, mother, grandmother, and wandering adventurer who left decades of grown-up life on the East Coast at age sixty to return to the mountains, beaches, and rain of her soul's home in the Pacific Northwest. She blogs about her adventures from coffee shops, her father's desk, national park lodges, her tent—wherever she feels cozy. She lives with her cat Lena in her family home in a small town in Washington—the real one.

Find resources for caregivers, book club guide, deleted book scenes, blog posts about life after Mama, and more at www.gretchenstaebler.com.

To follow the author's adventures in the PNW, visit www.writing downthestory.com.